MW00535125

THE
CHELATION
REVOLUTION

THE
CHELATION
REVOLUTION

The Breakthrough Detox Therapy

GARY GREENBERG

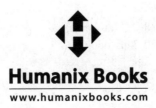

Humanix Books
www.humanixbooks.com

For Nomi, still the prettiest mom in the world

———————

Contents

Foreword

Tammy Born Huizenga, D.O.

When Gary Greenberg interviewed me about chelation therapy for a Newsmax magazine article, I told him he should come to my clinic in Grand Rapids, Michigan, to experience an integrative approach to medicine, see what we do and speak to some of our patients. His deadline for the article was too tight for him to take a trip from his home in South Florida, but he mentioned that he'd also been asked to write a book about chelation.

"Maybe I can come up for that project," he said. "I'll contact you after I sign the contract."

A few months later, contract presumably signed, he came to "embed himself" in the Born Clinic for a week, not only to see our facility and interview patients but also to experience chelation therapy himself. I invited him here because I am very proud of what we do in helping people achieve and maintain the best health possible. It is exciting to change lives for the better, and chelation is an integral part of that process for many of our patients.

Gary hung out here for a week, talking with patients and my staff. I believe the experience deepened his understanding of what chelation therapy can do for people and the type of care we offer to support our patients' health and well-being.

When I was in medical school, I was assigned to follow Dr. Grant Born at his office. His family practice focused on integrative medicine because he, himself, had experienced a heart problem called cardiomyopathy. His condition propelled him to look into alternative therapies because there were no conventional options for him other than having a heart transplant. When he began to feel better due to nutrition and chelation therapies, he knew he had to offer these same opportunities for healing to his patients.

After I graduated medical school, I joined Grant at his practice, and we were married five months later. Sadly, he died in 1998 due to a heart arrhythmia. It was sixteen years after his first diagnosis, despite initially being given just two years to live. We had worked together for eleven of those years growing an integrative practice, and we had recently moved into a state-of-the-art 22,000-square-foot clinic in southeast Grand Rapids when he passed away.

Since then, I've done my best to build upon what Grant started. He was always a proponent of chelation as a vital tool in helping people optimize their health. The key lies in its unique ability to reduce the load of toxic heavy metals that we all carry around in our bodies. In the modern industrialized world, it's virtually impossible to avoid accumulating some level of heavy-metal contamination. The most common and destructive offenders—lead, mercury, cadmium, arsenic, and aluminum—have no biological role in the human body but can disrupt cellular function, eventually contributing to chronic ailments such as heart disease, cancer, and dementia. There's no good reason to have these toxic substances in our bodies. Chelation therapy has been proven to be a safe and effective way to reduce levels of toxins and positively impact health.

It's important to note that chelation is not a magic bullet to cure all diseases, but rather an essential tool in helping the body function the way it was designed to function, which includes repairing and healing itself. At the Born Clinic, we offer a variety of therapies all working together to achieve that goal. We strive to identify and correct the root causes of problems rather than just treating symptoms with medications. We believe it's also important to educate patients about the causes of their conditions. Treatments are individualized, and we guide patients throughout the process. While chelation is not a universal panacea, it's hard to achieve better health with heavy metals lurking in tissues, continuously sabotaging various biological processes.

Those of us who use chelation for our patients (and ourselves) are confounded by the ongoing and often vehement resistance to the therapy by the conventional medical community. But I believe the tide is beginning to turn with compelling new research. My sincerest hopes are that this book will help to bring chelation out of the shadows and into the public consciousness. Our motto at the clinic is, "You were born to be healthy," and as you will see in the following pages, chelation therapy helps to remove a key impediment to the natural process of healing from many diseases for many patients.

Introduction

In this book, you will hear from some of the nation's leading chelation practitioners and their patients, who have experienced the therapy, which removes heavy metals from the tissue where they can reside for decades. Unless otherwise noted, all of their comments were told directly to me. Although everyone interviewed agreed to participate under their full names, to protect the patients' privacy we're only using their first name and last name initial. Chelation's practitioners uniformly stress that it is just part of a holistic treatment program, because achieving and maintaining good health goes beyond any one therapy, no matter how vital it is.

I owe the doctors and patients I interviewed an enormous debt of gratitude for candidly sharing with me their stories and resources. Like me, I'm sure they hope that the information on these pages will open your eyes to the health risks associated with even low-level heavy-metal contamination, and how chelation can help restore vitality to your body. After all, it's the only body you've got, and you're going to need it for a while.

CHAPTER 1

Meet Dr. Lamas

In some ways, the story of chelation is a mystery. For how can a therapy that has profoundly helped thousands upon thousands of people—many with hopeless health problems—be continuously and vehemently condemned by the conventional medical establishment?

Chelation's unique ability to remove heavy metals from the body offers holistic health benefits because these toxic substances contribute to the cell dysfunction that lies at the root of all degenerative diseases. And the success of chelation therapy has been well-documented for nearly seventy years. This includes relieving chest pain from heart disease, improving vision in people with macular degeneration, cutting through the fog of dementia, bringing the gangrenous limbs of diabetics back to life, helping to banish cancer and more. Yet chelation is still routinely branded as dangerous and ineffective, despite massive evidence to the contrary.

"The more I get into this, the more puzzled I am," says eminent cardiologist Dr. Gervasio Lamas, who has studied the therapy with the kind of thorough scientific methodology his peers demand. In the face of scathing criticism from the medical establishment, Lamas has stood firm to become chelation's most unlikely champion.

It's also a mystery why so few people have heard about chelation. Mention it to friends and family, and you're likely to be met with a blank stare. This holds true with generally well-educated, well-read folks, and even some in the medical field. That is an impressive degree of ignorance, especially considering the fact that chelation therapy has been around since the 1950s, and well over 100,000 Americans now undergo treatment every year.

If you ask your doctor about chelation, chances are good he or she will tell you that if you don't have lead poisoning or some other acute heavy-metal toxicity, you don't need it. The doctor will likely add that anyone who says it can help your health by ridding your body of low levels of heavy metals, or improve circulation in people with cardiovascular conditions, or benefit any other chronic health issue, is a quack at best or a charlatan at worst.

Dr. Lamas himself used to feel that way. He's the Chairman of Medicine and Chief of the Columbia University Division of Cardiology at Mount Sinai Medical Center in Miami Beach, and about as mainstream as medical doctors come. Called "Tony" by his pals, he graduated *cum laude* from Harvard University, earned his medical degree with honors from New York University, and completed his internship, residency, and cardiology training at Harvard Medical School's Brigham and Women's Hospital. There, he was known as "the pacemaker guy," because he focused on investigating the devices that treat heart arrhythmias. One of the trials he originated and directed revolutionized the way cardiologists use pacemakers.

One day in 1999, a new heart patient in Miami Beach asked Lamas about chelation. The patient was scruffy-looking and reminded the doctor of the TV detective Columbo, who typically asked a lot of seemingly inane questions that threw the perpetrators off guard, then tripped them up through his well-disguised guile and their own arrogance.

"I told him that chelation was quackery," recalls Lamas. "I said that it's expensive, it might be dangerous, and it's not going to help you."

That was the conventional medical community's standard chelation line, but "Columbo's" question nagged Lamas.

"As I thought about it, I realized that I was reacting to dogma, not data," he admits.

That dogma is pretty much set in stone. The Centers for Disease Control and Prevention (CDC), the U.S. Food and Drug Administration (FDA), the National Institutes of Health (NIH), the American Medical Association (AMA), and the American Heart Association (AHA) are among the prestigious groups contending that there is no substantial scientific evidence to support chelation therapy as an effective treatment for any medical condition other than acute heavy-metal poisoning. Potential risks are said to include kidney damage, irregular heartbeat, bone damage, loss of vitamins and minerals, and death.

Lamas started searching for data to support the medical community's pronouncements about chelation. Numerous observational studies and patient case histories reported by clinicians strongly suggested it was beneficial. Most notably, among other things, it seemed to banish chest pain from angina pectoris and improve circulation in the extremities of diabetics.

On the other hand, a few small placebo-controlled studies by cardiologists concluded it didn't do anything at all. The bottom line was that there were no reliable data to definitively say exactly what chelation did—good or bad—to the human body. So, Lamas went out and procured a $31.6 million grant from the NIH to fund a large, randomized, double-blind, placebo-controlled, "gold standard" study focused on heart disease patients that he dubbed the Trial to Access Chelation Therapy (TACT).

Surely, Lamas thought, TACT would settle the chelation controversy once and for all. But it didn't quite work out that way, which is one reason it remains a pariah therapy and why so many people still have never heard of it.

PHYSICIAN PROFILE
DR. GERVASIO "TONY" LAMAS

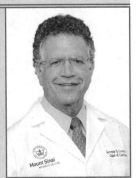

Chairman of Medicine and Chief of
the Columbia University Division
of Cardiology, Mount Sinai Medical
Center, Miami Beach, Florida
Undergraduate: Harvard College,
Biochemical Sciences, 1974
Medical School: New York University,
1978
Specialty: Cardiology
Selected Honors and Associations:

- Fellow of the American College of
  Cardiology
- Fellow of the American Heart Association
- Fellow of the European Society of Cardiology
- Former Chairman of the Clinical Trials Review Committee of
  the National Heart, Lung and Blood Institute
- Past President of the South Florida American Heart
  Association
- Originated and served as chairman of the Mode Selection
  Trial (MOST) in Sinus Node Dysfunction that revolutionized
  cardiac pacemaker functionality
- Co-Chair of the Occluded Artery Trial (OAT)
- Originated and served as study chair for the Trial to Assess
  Chelation Therapy (TACT)
- Published more than 200 peer-reviewed articles and over
  150 abstracts in medical journals, including the *New England
  Journal of Medicine*, the *Journal of the American Medical
  Association*, *Annals of Internal Medicine*, *Circulation*, and
  the *Journal of the American College of Cardiology*.

Website: www.msmc.com/doctor/gervasio-a-lamas-2

Quote: "I think we are nearing the end of the beginning, but
we are far from the beginning of the end in showing that EDTA
should be used for patients with severe vascular disease. These
are exciting times. For me, it's become a labor of love."

CHAPTER 2

The Landmark TACT Study: Chelation Moves into the Mainstream

The undertaking of the TACT study was a herculean effort, and Dr. Tony Lamas was likely one of just a handful of people in the world who could have pulled it off, thanks to his vast experience originating and conducting scientific studies, his brilliance in both research and clinical medicine, and, appropriately, his "tact" to bridge both the conventional and alternative medical communities.

No doubt his wry sense of humor also helped. When asked in a 2019 interview why a traditionally trained cardiologist would spend so much of his professional career focused on an "alternative" therapy, he chuckled and replied: "I was asking myself that same question in the bathroom mirror this morning."

First, Lamas had to gain the trust of a wary chelation community, because he needed the help of seasoned practitioners to treat 1,700-plus patients with dozens of infusions each in a study that would take years to complete. In the past, many of the practitioners—mostly doctors of osteopathy and integrative

MDs—felt persecuted by the medical establishment. They'd been harried, discredited, sued, and even run out of the country.

Dr. Robert Willix, a former heart surgeon who owned a chelation clinic in Boca Raton, Florida, in the late 1980s, says, "Chelation is very powerful and helped a lot of people but was always on the fringe, so you had to watch what you were doing. The powers that be put pressure on practitioners, investigating them for not practicing traditional medicine. The standard of care for coronary artery disease was bypass surgery and stents. If you started doing chelation on people who could get a stent or bypass, your waiting room would fill with lawyers."

Some practitioners feared Lamas was out to prove that chelation was, indeed, quackery, and that he would shade or interpret data to reach a foregone conclusion. If that happened, the study could leave them worse off than they were. Despite the headwinds they faced from the medical establishment, at least they were able to practice the therapy before TACT.

A bad outcome would put more pressure on them and perhaps even limit their ability to use the therapy. And if the results were undeniably positive, mainstream doctors and the insurance industry would possibly embrace chelation and create enough competition, regulations, and payment caps to make their lives more difficult or even drive them out of business.

Lamas also had to figure out how best to isolate the chelation part of the standard therapy, which is a holistic approach that typically includes vitamin and mineral supplements along with other complementary modalities and lifestyle changes. If he didn't totally isolate the chelation, critics could point out that other factors may be responsible for any improvements.

If he did isolate the chelation, it may not prove as effective as possible, or it could even trigger other problems, because some of

TACT (Trial to Assess Chelation Therapy)

SCOPE: Placebo-controlled, double-blind design that included 1,708 participants aged 50 years and older with a prior heart attack.
PURPOSE: To test whether EDTA chelation therapy and/or high-dose vitamin therapy is effective for the treatment of coronary heart disease.
FINDINGS: Those receiving chelation had an 18% reduced risk of subsequent cardiac events such as heart attack, stroke, hospitalization for angina, or coronary revascularization. A cardiac event occurred in 222 (26%) of the chelation group and 261 (30%) of the placebo group.
DIABETES SUB-GROUP: People with diabetes made up 37% of the total group. Death from any cause was 43% lower in those patients with diabetes who received chelation.

the substances chelation removes are beneficial and need to be replaced via supplements.

There was also no standard as to the ideal number of EDTA infusions for treatment of coronary artery disease (CAD), the subject of the TACT study. Some very sick patients needed as many as a hundred infusions, or more, to show a marked improvement, while others needed as few as twenty, or less. And how would they measure chelation's effects? Should they focus on hard objective data, such as future cardiac events and deaths, or choose more interpretive items such as scans, stress tests, and coronary artery calcium numbers?

Perhaps the biggest hurdle was finding enough volunteers who fit the specs. They had to have some degree of heart disease, but people who were relatively healthy may not have shown as much of a change as those who were sicker. And people with really diseased coronary arteries may have been too far along for chelation to help over a limited timeframe. Lamas also had to find enough people willing to undergo many months of time-consuming infusions with just a fifty-fifty chance of actually getting the drug that may, or may not, help their condition.

Needless to say, it was a daunting task. And that's before you even get to the administrative side of responsibly doling out more than $30 million.

"It's really like putting together a small business organization," says Lamas. "And every piece of the puzzle has to have the goal of scientific clarity and validity. If it's not scientifically valid, you don't do it.

"I had behind me the very best academic clinical research organization in the world, the Duke Clinical Research Institute. I also have superb people working with me on the administration end of it. Basically, it's just me, my research manager, and three people working under her, but we get a tremendous amount of work done. If this were a large-scale pharmaceutical trial, what we do would have a staff of thirty, or more."

In the end, Lamas and his team amassed 134 testing sites split fairly evenly between chelation practitioners at alternative or complementary clinics and institutions such as university hospitals and cardiology research centers. They chose participants who were over the age of fifty and had suffered at least one heart attack more than six weeks previously. They decided to do forty infusions on each—thirty weekly and another ten monthly—which some practitioners feared wouldn't be enough to demonstrate the treatment's true potential. Then they broke the participants into four groups—EDTA infusions with supplements, EDTA infusions with placebo supplements, placebo infusions with supplements, and placebo infusions with placebo supplements—and got under way.

Historical Headwinds

Beyond the practical side of putting together TACT, Lamas was bucking a firmly established bias against chelation by his peers in the conventional medical community. It is at the core of the chelation mystery, as little in its history validates such vitriol.

Derived from the Greek word *chele*, meaning "claw," chelation is the ability of certain compounds to latch onto mineral and metal ions. When used in the body, chelation can pull lead, mercury, arsenic, cadmium and other harmful heavy metals out of the tissues in which they have settled and into the bloodstream, where they are processed and eliminated, mainly in urine through the kidneys and urinary tract.

These compounds, called "chelates" or "chelators," were first utilized practically in industry to remove heavy metals and minerals during the production of various products, including paints and textiles. In 1935, the Germans filed a patent for the chelating agent ethylenediaminetetraacetic acid (EDTA), a synthetic amino acid which was used to extract calcium from water used in the dye-making process, thus stabilizing colors.

A few years later, Georgetown University biochemistry professor Martin Rubin found that EDTA's metal- and calcium-binding properties could be used medically. Among other things, it inhibited blood clotting, and it is still widely used today as an anticoagulant in the purple-topped collection tubes you may see at your doctor's office when you go for a blood test.

In the 1950s, Detroit physician Dr. Norman Clarke Sr. started using intravenous EDTA to treat car battery factory workers for lead poisoning. Surprisingly, the infusions also seemed to relieve symptoms of angina pectoris, a heart condition that causes chest pain due to constricted coronary arteries. His patients with heart disease needed less nitroglycerin to dilate the coronary arteries and could do more physically before feeling chest pain. So Clarke decided to try EDTA on his heart patients who weren't suffering from lead poisoning.

Between 1956 and 1960, Clarke and his team treated 283 heart patients with intravenous EDTA, and 87 percent of them reported reduced symptoms. By the way, Clarke was no wild-eyed alternative medicine revolutionary bent on overthrowing the medical establishment. He was a well-respected researcher and innovator who authored a variety of scientific papers in addition to those on chelation. He also brought the first privately-owned electrocardiograph machine to Detroit and stayed in active practice until the ripe old age of eighty-seven.

There are several types of EDTA, and they have different properties. For instance, potassium EDTA is the version used as an anticoagulant in the purple-topped blood collection bottles. Clarke employed disodium EDTA to treat heart patients, and that is the most common drug used by practitioners today.

One drawback of disodium EDTA is that infusing too much, too fast can potentially cause kidney damage and other problems. Researchers figured this out in the 1950s and developed safe treatment protocols. Still, there have been fatalities due to improper administration of the drug, and those few cases are cited over and over again by chelation opponents in warnings about the dangers of the therapy.

Despite resistance from the establishment, chelation practitioners pressed on, and in 1973 the American Institute of Medical Preventics was formed to promote the therapy as well as train and certify practitioners. The organization later changed its name to the American College for Advancement of Medicine (ACAM) and remains chelation's most prominent training resource and institutional advocate.

Meanwhile, several studies were performed with almost uniformly positive results, but they were primarily observational with a limited number of participants—and summarily dismissed by chelation critics.

Doctors Ray Evers and Carlos Lamar amassed volumes of anecdotal evidence that EDTA chelation improved circulation, in some cases saving gangrenous limbs of diabetics suffering from peripheral artery disease. Evers was eventually sued by the FDA for using chelation drugs—which were FDA-approved only for heavy metal detoxification—to treat cardiovascular conditions. In 1981, he won a landmark legal case, setting a precedent allowing doctors to use any FDA-approved drug "off-label" at their own discretion, a common practice today.

One of the most jaw-dropping studies was performed by Scandinavian doctors Claus Hancke and Knut Flytlie. It involved ninety-two patients who were on waiting lists for either heart bypass operations or limb amputations due to vascular issues. After chelation therapy for an average of six months, the doctors reported that fifty-eight of the sixty-five bypass patients were able to cancel their surgery, and the same held true for twenty-four of the twenty-seven awaiting amputation.

A follow-up study years later on forty-seven of the heart patients found that thirty-four of them still hadn't had surgical intervention. In 1992, integrative physician Dr. Jonathan Collin remarked: "If we extrapolate these numbers to the large number of bypass surgeries and amputations performed in the United States, 363,000 of the 407,000 bypass surgeries may have been avoided and 102,000 limbs may have been saved if chelation therapy had been administered to these patients. Furthermore, $8 billion in health care costs may have been saved."

Despite a plethora of anecdotal and clinical evidence that chelation could indeed work miracles for some patients, there remained a lack of definitive proof in the form of a large, randomized, placebo-controlled, double-blind study. That shortcoming fueled attacks by the medical establishment, including legal assaults that threatened the licenses and livelihood of practitioners.

Some of the most vicious attacks against chelation were carried out by a band of medical doctors and others who call themselves "Skeptics" but are commonly known as "The Quackbusters." Through internet websites, media outlets and legal proceedings, they strive to root out fraudulent medical practices. That's not necessarily a bad thing, as there are plenty of unscrupulous people around who take advantage of the desperate and ill-informed with bogus products and therapies. But the Quackbusters tend to target all kinds of alternative practitioners indiscriminately, often in a dismissive, ridiculing manner (see sidebar in Chapter 4).

With chelation therapy saddled by a long-ingrained resistance fueled in part by the media-savvy Quackbusters, only a bona fide gold standard study could possibly quiet the critics and convince the mainstream medical community to give it some respect. And that brings us back to Dr. Tony Lamas and his gutsy pursuit of the truth.

TACT Stirs the Pot

TACT came under attack long before any results were in. In 2008, a group led by retired anesthesiologist and Quackbuster Dr. Kimball C. Atwood IV penned an article in *The Medscape Journal of Medicine* titled "Why the NIH Trial to Assess Chelation Therapy (TACT) Should Be Abandoned." The fifty-one-page article blasted TACT as "unethical, dangerous, pointless and wasteful."

The article sparked a probe by the U.S. Office of Human Research Protections, the federal agency required by law to investigate all allegations of human subject violations in research. While the claims were being checked out, recruitment of new patients for the TACT study was suspended.

In defending TACT, Beth Clay, a former senior professional staff member of the U.S. House of Representatives Committee on Government Reform, wrote a lengthy article in *The Journal of American Physicians and Surgeons*. She noted that Atwood and his co-authors admitted being "a tiny but shrill minority of physicians," and she warned that "abandonment of this research could result in denial of a potentially life-saving therapy to many patients."

Clay also called Atwood and his fellow authors "unqualified" and "biased," and pointed out they had conflicts of interests because some of them derived income from legal compensation for testifying in cases against alternative medicine practitioners. In the end, TACT was delayed about a year before it was exonerated. It finally concluded in 2011.

TACT Results

In 2012, the study became unblinded, and the results that had been tallied by leading statisticians at Duke University and scrutinized by a clinical events committee from Harvard University finally came to light.

Lamas, who'd initially thought that TACT would put chelation practitioners out of business, remembers the moment of discovery distinctly.

"We opened the book—five of us in the leadership of investigators—at a long table at Duke and, by God, the darn thing is positive," he recalls during an interview with podcaster Kirk Hamilton. "We were able to reduce a combined clinical endpoint, which means for either death, heart attack, stroke, bypass or angioplasty, and hospitalization for unstable angina, and that was in all comers with a heart attack.

"That's a spectacular result. If this stuff had been a statin drug you'd be calling me in Paris, and I'd be sipping champagne."

Specifically, there was an 18 percent overall reduction of cardiovascular events and death from any cause in the active group versus those taking the placebo chelation. That is a minimally significant benefit. But about one-third of the patients were diabetic, and in that subgroup, the results were far more dramatic.

"In those patients, chelation reduced the risk of the combined cardiovascular endpoint by 41 percent," says Lamas. "That's extraordinary. It reduced the risk of death from all causes over five years by 43 percent, and it reduced the risk of another heart attack by just over 50 percent."

So, finally, chelation practitioners had definitive scientific proof in a gold-standard study that chelation helped all heart patients to some degree and diabetics quite a lot. And it was very safe, because in performing 55,222 infusions there were just a handful of adverse reactions—most very minor—with slightly more in the placebo group. There was also one death in each group that may or may not have been related to the infusions.

Still, Lamas and his fellow authors conservatively concluded that the results "provide evidence to guide further research but are not sufficient to support the routine use of chelation therapy."

When the TACT results appeared in the prestigious *Journal of the American Medical Association (JAMA)*, it was like poking a hornet's nest. A buzzing swarm of criticism from the medical establishment was unleashed, and even *JAMA* came under fire for having the audacity to publish the study. The editors took the unprecedented step of writing a letter to defend their decision, noting that TACT underwent considerably more scrutiny than most studies that are run in the journal.

They also said: "The decision to publish was related to the investigators, who include one of the most preeminent cardiovascular researchers (Lamas) and one of the most respected statisticians (Duke University's Kerry Lee, Ph.D.)."

In the same issue, *JAMA* editors also ran a scathing companion editorial by the Cleveland Clinic's Dr. Steven Nissen. He noted the relatively high drop-out rate of study subjects, with considerably more from the placebo group. Nissen surmised that they may have dropped out because they were made aware they were on the placebo, thus "unmasking" the supposedly blind study and compromising its findings.

He also took issue with the inclusion of two "less reliable endpoints" in cardiac revascularization (stents and bypasses) and hospitalization for angina. He claims those "soft endpoints" could have led to biased investigators pumping up those numbers in the placebo group to make chelation seem more effective than it was.

"The results cannot be accepted . . . and do not demonstrate a benefit for chelation," he concluded in the editorial.

Nissen seems particularly dismissive of the alternative or integrative medicine infusion sites. In a 2019 interview with *Newsmax* magazine, he branded the TACT study as "low quality, sloppy and poorly funded," adding, "The people doing this are one of the worst collections of quacks and alternative medicine folks who don't practice scientific-based medicine."

Ironically, the non-alternative medicine testing sites, which were largely cardiology practices, had more positive results for chelation than the alternative sites.

Nissen appears to be most concerned that chelation could divert some patients from getting heart bypass operations, stents, and other standard therapies. When asked to be interviewed for this book, Nissen declined because he felt the book would be promoting chelation, which he said is "extremely dangerous to public health."

Following the publication of the TACT results, many cardiologists and other MDs joined Nissen on the anti-chelation bandwagon. Dr. Valentin Fuster, past president of the American Heart Association, declared, "The whole list of statistics was very borderline." That directly contradicted TACT statistician

Kerry Lee, who is widely regarded to be the leading biomedical statistician in the world. And on *The Cardiology Show with Dr. Fuster*, Dr. Clyde Yancy, Chief of the Division of Cardiology at Northwestern University Feinberg School of Medicine, summed up the general consensus of the expert panelists by saying: "We need to pause to really put this in context. . . . My own feeling is that we should pause indefinitely."

But some of their more open-minded colleagues defended the study.

"Back in 2003, when this trial was announced, I thought it was a crazy notion," Dr. Eric Topol, a cardiologist with the Scripps Translational Science Institute in San Diego, wrote in an article for Medscape.com. "At the end of the day, after all this work of all these investigators, I give them credit. And I give the *JAMA* editors credit for publishing it."

And in an editorial in the journal *Circulation: Cardiovascular Quality and Outcomes*, Dr. Sanjay Kaul, a cardiologist at Cedars-Sinai Medical Center in Los Angeles, concludes: "Although the debate surrounding TACT is clearly warranted, the arguments that the TACT results are not valid or reliable are overstated. Consequently, the calls for a hasty dismissal are unfair and undoubtedly unjustified."

So, despite Lamas' extraordinary efforts on TACT, the jury is still out on chelation.

"I presented the data to the FDA in 2014, and asked that the drug be approved for cardiovascular disease," recalls Lamas. "They said, 'The study is positive. The drug is safe. But it is only one study. You need to do it again.'

"At that point, I realized I was caught in another ten-year vortex."

Thus, TACT 2 was born. In September 2016, it was announced that the NIH and the National Center for Complementary and

Integrative Health (NCCIH) put up $37 million to fund the trial. This time, the scope is narrower, with the focus on type 2 diabetics only.

"The requirement of proof is so strict it takes a lot to show that something works," says Lamas. "A lot of money too. The TACT studies are close to $100 million now, and nobody is going to make a billion dollars on this because the drug is long out of patent. You won't see a pharmaceutical company supporting it, and you'll never see an ad for it on TV."

Lamas makes clear his goal is not to prove chelation is a miracle treatment for the myriad of maladies that its proponent have claimed. Instead he is focused on his speciality of cardiovascular diseases and wants to prove or disprove its efficacy as a life-saving treatment for his patients.

Lamas hopes to have the results by sometime in early 2023. The goal is to show that EDTA is both safe and effective so that the FDA will approve it for the treatment of cardiovascular disease. If approved, chelation therapy will not only gain legitimacy for this purpose but also more likely be eligible for insurance coverage. Currently, it is an out-of-pocket expense, and a series of treatments typically runs thousands of dollars.

Lamas has something else up his sleeve and has launched a TACT 3a trial, which we'll discuss in an upcoming chapter.

Meanwhile, the once-skeptical cardiologist has made chelation somewhat of a crusade.

"Chelation practitioners have been persecuted for decades, and I do not understand at what point the hatred and bias against chelation made good scientists unable to look at our data objectively," says Lamas, supporting his case by rattling off the credentials of his team. "I have been doing this for a while and have a good reputation as a clinical trialist. My lead statistician, Dr. Kerry Lee, is probably the most respected biostatistician in the world, and I had my event adjudicated at Harvard Brigham and Women's. So I had the best people all the way through the process. And then we present our findings, and they say, 'You got the wrong answer, boy.'"

But Lamas isn't giving up anytime soon. He's not only continuing with the TACT studies but also serves as a one-man awareness campaign. He's lectured to thousands of physicians about chelation, and he feels that the tide is finally beginning to turn for the "pariah therapy."

"They used to think that chelation was just a wacky, even dangerous, idea," he says. "Now, they think there could be something interesting here. They have gone from rabid atheists to agnostics. It's TACT 2 that will get them into church. That's why it's so important."

CHAPTER 3

You Were Born to Be Healthy

Inside the Born Clinic

On a surprisingly chilly October morning in Grand Rapids, Michigan, I Uber from my hotel by the airport to the Born Clinic. I've come here to research this book about chelation, an underappreciated therapy that not only reduces the concentration of toxic heavy metals in the body but also seems to rejuvenate the circulatory system, which can affect all aspects of health.

As I walk into the Born Clinic, the morning chill quickly dissipates, not only from the change of temperature inside but also by the inviting atmosphere. Although the lobby/waiting room is cavernous, with a domed ceiling, it still feels homey, with a fireplace, a smattering of upholstered furniture with throw pillows, and fish tanks. Soothing New Age music plays in the background, and on the wall facing the entranceway are large backlit letters with the clinic's motto:

"YOU WERE BORN TO BE HEALTHY."

The morning IV session crowd has already begun to congregate in this serene haven from the outside world. Most are here for chelation infusions. While waiting to be called, some patients chat amongst themselves, others read, work on laptops, or just stare at the cell phone in their palm. I settle in at a small hightop table next to one of the two fish tanks. In the week that I've been here, this has become my favorite spot to write when I'm not otherwise occupied interviewing patients and staff, or undergoing chelation infusions myself.

But I barely have time to fire up my laptop and check my email before I'm introduced to Robert and Marilyn Morris, who are sitting by the fireplace and have volunteered to be interviewed for my book. They've been coming here since 1996, when Marilyn suddenly began feeling fatigued.

"I was so tired I'd go downstairs and put the laundry in, and I had to sit for a while before I had enough energy to climb the stairs," she says. "And then I started feeling like I had a ton of bricks on my chest."

Meanwhile, Robert had a client at his real estate agency who had suffered a heart attack and was told she needed a triple bypass operation. Instead, she opted for chelation at the Born Clinic.

"Her heart doctor in Kalamazoo warned her that chelation was snake oil," says Robert. "Then, after having thirty-some chelation treatments, she went back to see him and had a stress test. The doctor told her, 'I can't believe it. Your heart is fine. What did you do?' And she told him, 'I went up to Grand Rapids and got some of that snake oil.'"

It turned out that both Marilyn and Robert needed chelation therapy, she for her three clogged coronary arteries and he for plaque buildup in the carotids, which supply blood to the brain.

"I was a stroke victim waiting to happen and had twenty treatments," says Robert. "Marilyn needed forty, but she started feeling really well somewhere in the thirties. The advantage was she didn't need bypass surgery and all the rehab that goes along with it. And she didn't have to go on any drugs."

That was more than twenty years ago, and she hasn't had any heart problems since.

"Robert wasn't so lucky," says Marilyn. "He had a heart attack last April."

Robert grunts. "It wasn't really a heart attack in the normal sense," he explains. "I was remodeling a house and a window frame fell on my foot. It caused a clot that traveled to my heart."

"That's a heart attack," Marilyn says with a smirk.

"But I don't have heart disease," he notes.

"Maybe not, but you did have a heart attack," Marilyn says, getting the last word in.

Robert laughs. After fifty-five years of marriage together, he knows when he can't win.

"In any case," he continues, "I went to a well-known heart doctor in St. Joseph and he said I had some blockage in a small artery. He wasn't going to do anything about it except give me medication that I'd probably have to take for life. So, I let Dr. Born handle it. I started breathing better after seven chelation treatments, and it took about twenty in all to get back to where I was."

Robert and Marilyn have been regulars at the clinic for more than two decades. Mostly, that's been for maintenance, which works out to once-a-month chelation infusions. They've seen a lot here over the years.

"One guy was sitting here white as a sheet because his doctor had given him just a few weeks to live," says Robert. "After two or three months of chelation, I saw him not crawling or shuffling or even walking out of here. He was running and looked twenty-five years younger.

"We've seen so many miracles at this place, and I know neither one of us would be here now without major surgeries. All our friends who laughed at us for coming here are gone, mostly from heart attacks and strokes."

Robert is not only still here at age seventy-six, but hale and hearty and working. Along with his real estate agency, he has a construction business.

"My dad was a migrant worker, and one day when he was working in the cotton fields of Missouri, he woke me up and said, 'It's five o'clock in the morning, you're five years old, and it's time to get to work," he recalls. "I've been working ever since."

Robert and Marilyn wish me luck with my book, and head off. A few minutes later, I'm called for my chelation session by Liza Ewing, a licensed practical nurse who serves as the supervisor of the clinic's IV Therapy Department. The infusion room is nearly as large as the lobby, with floor-to-ceiling windows offering a panoramic view of the suburban countryside. Liza sits me down, asks which arm I prefer being punctured, and compliments me on my well-defined veins.

IV nurses are a unique breed. They tend to be friendly, chatty, and compassionate. Yet their expertise lies in sticking people, and it's likely they wouldn't have gone into that particular specialty if they didn't enjoy it. Or maybe they just enjoy trying to make the process as painless as possible.

"Just a little pinch," Liza says as she slides the IV needle into a prominent vein on the topside of my left forearm.

I barely feel it. Liza is originally from Texas, and I joke about her being a Ewing, as in J.R. of the *Dallas* TV show fame. No doubt she's heard it before, but laughs politely. She's been working at the Born Clinic for sixteen years, but she's still got a bit of Texas twang in her voice.

"What chelation case most sticks in your mind?" I ask her.

She ponders the question for just a few seconds before saying: "An elderly gentleman in his nineties came in here in a wheelchair with a foot that was bluish, blackish, and purplish. He had pretty severe vascular disease, and his doctors had told him his foot would have to be amputated. Several months into chelation, he was walking on that foot. A few years later, I was invited to his 100th birthday party, and I danced with him at that party.

"I think that left such a lasting impression because I'd only been working here for a little while and was pretty new to this field. I didn't really know what I thought about this type of treatment, and that was a real eye-opener for me."

Liza anchors down my IV needle with a transparent adhesive patch and escorts me and my IV pole to one of the two dozen or so plush leather recliners scattered about the room. As I settle in, she introduces me to my neighbor. He's an elderly gentleman who's so relaxed he seems to be half-melted into the recliner. He perks up once we start chatting, and another life-altering chelation story begins to unfurl.

Roman Rabiej tells me he's seventy-nine-and-a-half years old and was a professor of engineering for fifty of those years. He started in his native Poland and wound up at Western Michigan University, but he developed some serious cardiovascular issues along the way. In the mid-1990s, a cardiologist told him he needed a heart bypass operation.

"My wife and I read Dr. Dean Ornich's book (*Program for Reversing Heart Disease*) and told the doctor we wanted to try that," recalls Roman. "He said, 'I don't believe you can do that.' So I said, 'I don't believe you are a very good doctor.'"

Roman made the lifestyle changes recommended by Ornich and managed to go ten years before finally getting a stent in his left anterior descending artery, which is commonly called the "widow-maker."

His heart held up pretty well, but in 2015 he began feeling dizzy and had to hold onto his desk at times during class to keep from falling.

"After a while, I couldn't drive, and then I began forgetting things," he says. "One day I graded exams, but then couldn't remember what to do with the grades. I even forgot how to say the *Hail Mary*, which I'd been saying every day for all of my life. I was like a zombie. My wife had to take me by the hand and guide me around. I felt helpless."

He went to the hospital for an MRI and other tests, and was told he had a blockage in an artery at the base of his skull.

"They said it was too close to the brain for them to do anything, and they sent me home to die," he says with a chuckle. "They didn't actually say that, but that's how I interpreted it."

Meanwhile, his troubled circulatory system also caused intermittent claudication, a condition in which restricted blood flow to the legs causes excruciating pain when walking. Out of desperation, Roman's devoted wife followed the advice of friends and drove him to the Born Clinic, where he began chelation treatments.

"At this time, I was almost unable to read," he says. "Dr. Born told me that as soon as we improve the blood flow to my brain, it will clear up my mind."

He came to the clinic two to three times a week for chelation infusions. It took dozens of treatments, but the fog eventually began to lift and the pain in his legs subsided.

Within six months, Roman was back to driving and continued teaching until retiring in 2016. The following year, he suffered a massive heart attack. He says it wasn't from a typical blockage but rather the vessel collapsing where the stent had been placed more than a decade earlier.

"I didn't know I had a heart attack and walked around with it for a few days before the pain got too bad," he says. "I needed a six-hour operation, but the surgeon did a good job, because I'm alive. After three weeks, I stopped using pharmaceutical drugs. I took vitamins and minerals and continued to come here for chelation treatments one or two times a month. Two years have passed, and I'm in good shape. I never felt better."

The man who could barely walk a block a few years ago now uses his cell phone's pedometer function and racks up as many as 25,000 steps a day. And the man who couldn't think straight now regularly wins chess matches against his son, who has multiple post-graduate degrees and works as a project manager for Google.

"Dr. Born gave me back my life," he says. "Maybe I would still be here, but what kind of life is it when you can't think or walk?"

By the time Roman finishes telling me his story, his IV bag is drained of the yellow chelating fluid. He takes off, looking spry with a bounce in his step. I just sit here relaxing, thinking about all I've seen and heard in the past week, and how to capture it in words. As the last few CCs in my bag drip down and flow through the tubing and needle into my vein, I feel pretty good. My energy level is up, and whatever remnant of beer-imbibing brain fog I might have had when I got here a couple of hours ago is completely gone.

You've got to wonder how something that seems to help so many can continue to be shunned by most doctors and remain unknown to most people. Hopefully, that's all about to change.

IN THEIR OWN WORDS

My wife had stomach cancer but didn't want chemo so she was treated in Mexico, and that's where I first heard about chelation. Now, Dr. Born treats her, and when we come here, I do chelation. At first, I had a bug in my intestines that caused constant diarrhea. Turns out I was allergic to gluten and also had high levels of lead, cadmium, and aluminum. I cut gluten out of my diet and was treated for heavy metals, and that bug went away. I'd also been fighting gout for years, but the medication I took had side effects. Dr. Born gave me a natural supplement, and that and the chelation took care of my gout. Getting those metals out of my body made me feel better, and I have more energy. Conventional doctors think chelation and supplements are funny stuff, but when you sit here and talk to all these people and see how much chelation and these other things help them, you realize that what the conventional doctors do with all their drugs is the funny stuff.

Donald B., 82, Bay City, Michigan

PHYSICIAN PROFILE
DR. TAMMY BORN HUIZENGA

The Born Clinic, Grand Rapids, Michigan

Undergraduate: Calvin College, Science & Chemistry, 1982

Medical School: Michigan State University College of Osteopathic Medicine, 1986

Specialty: Integrative family medicine

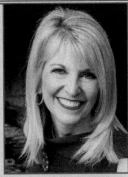

Photo credit: Kelly Braman Photography

Selected Honors and Associations:

- Testified before the U.S. Congressional House Committee of Government Reform regarding the Freedom of Medical Access Bill in 1998.
- Past president of the Michigan Board of Osteopathic Medicine and Surgery
- Served on the Medicare Coverage Advisory Committee and the Advisory Committee on Training in Primary Care Medicine and Dentistry Health Resources and Services Administration during the George W. Bush presidency
- Appointed to National Advisory Council for Complementary and Integrative Health in 2018

Website: https://bornclinic.com

Quote: "Depending on genetics and other factors, some people can handle far less heavy-metal contamination than others. But there's no good reason to have heavy metals in our bodies. Why not get those metals out?"

CHAPTER 4

From Lead Poisoning to Heart Disease and Beyond

D r. Robert Battle first heard about chelation therapy in the mid-1960s when he was a young family physician fresh out of medical school. He read an article written about the Ford Hospital in Detroit using intravenous chelation to treat kids for lead poisoning.

"Children were having seizures caused by lead intoxication from the auto-battery factories and their lead smelters near where they lived," says Battle. "It caused an epidemic of reduced efficiency in the educational process, plummeting SAT scores, and a general dumbing down."

When the parents saw their children's improvement after chelation treatments, they started trying it themselves for various health problems and found that it helped cardiovascular conditions to the point that some were able to ditch their medications.

Excited about the potential of chelation therapy in treating cardiovascular disease, Battle brought the article to a staff meeting at the hospital where he worked.

"My colleagues treated me like a leper and said if I planned to keep my license, I better never mention that dirty word 'chelation' again," recalls Battle. "I really didn't know any better, so I threw the article in the trash, thinking I'd been badly mistaken.

"For the next fifteen years, I practiced conventional medicine, even though I began to feel like I'd become a drug dealer for the pharmaceutical companies. Then I rediscovered chelation therapy, and it transformed my future."

The Basics

So what is chelation? A potentially life-altering therapy that can safely and effectively be used in the treatment of a variety of medical conditions, or a dangerous alternative medicine gimmick that is costly, ineffective, possibly harmful, and could prevent people from seeking conventional medical care?

The answer depends on who you ask. And there doesn't seem to be a lot of common ground beyond it providing treatment for heavy-metal toxicity. To better understand the divide, let's start with the basics.

Derived from the Greek word *chele*, meaning "claw," chelation is the ability of certain compounds to latch onto mineral and metal ions. When used in the body, chelation can pull lead, mercury, arsenic, cadmium, and other harmful heavy metals out of the tissues in which they have settled and into the bloodstream, where they are processed and eliminated, mainly in urine through the kidneys and urinary tract. These compounds, called chelates, were first theorized in 1892 by French-Swiss scientist Alfred Werner. He actually had a revelation about "coordination compounds" (the binding of organic and inorganic molecules) in a dream, and it eventually led to him winning the Nobel Prize for Chemistry in 1913. Ironically, Werner suffered from atherosclerosis—one of the conditions chelation therapy is reputed to help—and died at age fifty-three.

Werner's groundbreaking discovery was first utilized practically in industry to remove heavy metals and minerals during the production of various products, including paints and textiles. In 1935, the Germans filed a patent for the chelating agent ethylenediaminetetraacetic acid (EDTA), a synthetic amino acid that was used to extract calcium from water used in the dye-making process, thus stabilizing colors. During World War II, British chemists seeking an antidote for an arsenic-based chemical weapon found that EDTA was particularly effective in treating lead poisoning.

Around the same time, Georgetown University biochemistry professor Martin Rubin serendipitously heard about EDTA. One of his graduate students worked part-time for the FDA and met a man who was seeking approval of EDTA as a food additive to preserve color and freshness. While waiting to talk to officials, the man told the grad student, "One day, EDTA will be used to treat heart disease by removing calcium blockages in arteries." That tidbit of hearsay prompted Rubin to start studying EDTA. He found it did indeed possess metal- and calcium-binding properties, with one result being that it inhibited blood clotting. It is still widely used today as an anticoagulant in the purple-topped collection tubes you may see at your doctor's office when you go for a blood test.

In 1952, a young child, who'd apparently eaten some paint chips from a window sill, turned up at the Georgetown University Hospital emergency room with acute lead poisoning. Pediatrician Dr. S. P. Bessman knew of Rubin's work with EDTA and, with few options for helping the child, tried the desperate measure of using the chelating compound to get the lead out. It worked, and the case was reported in *Medical Annals, District of Columbia.*

When Detroit physician Dr. Norman Clarke, Sr., read the report, he started using intravenous EDTA to treat car battery factory workers for lead poisoning. Surprisingly, the infusions also seemed to relieve symptoms of angina pectoris, a heart condition that causes chest pain due to constricted coronary arteries. His patients with heart disease needed less nitroglycerin to dilate the coronary arteries and could do more physically before feeling chest pain. So, Clarke decided to try EDTA on his heart patients who weren't suffering from lead poisoning.

Between 1956 and 1960, Clarke and his team treated 283 heart patients with intravenous EDTA, and 87 percent of them reported reduced symptoms. Clarke initially theorized that the EDTA removed calcium from "hardened" coronary arteries, improving blood flow and relieving the trademark chest tightness of angina. He later came to believe that the calcium removal wasn't the primary factor in enhancing coronary circulation; rather, it was the removal of heavy metals that inhibit cell function and lower defenses to destructive free radicals. Both theories are still being debated today.

Clarke was no wild-eyed alternative medicine revolutionary bent on overthrowing the medical establishment. He was a well-respected researcher and innovator who authored a variety of scientific papers in addition to those on chelation. He also brought the first privately owned electrocardiograph machine to Detroit and stayed in active practice until the ripe old age of eighty-seven.

EDTA Chelation's Bumpy Ride

There are several types of EDTA, and they have different properties. For instance, potassium EDTA is the version used as an anticoagulant in the purple-topped blood collection bottles. Clarke employed disodium EDTA to treat heart patients, and that is the most common drug used by practitioners today. One drawback of disodium EDTA is that infusing too much too fast can potentially cause kidney damage and other problems. Researchers figured this out in the 1950s and developed safe treatment protocols. Still, there have been fatalities due to improper administration of the drug. Three high-profile cases in the early 2000s, involving the tragic deaths of two young children and an adult, continue to be cited by chelation opponents in warnings about the dangers of the therapy. Ironically, when administered properly, EDTA has been shown to actually improve kidney function when it is impaired by lead toxicity and some other medical conditions. Studies and reviews attesting to that benefit have been published in prestigious medical journals, including *Nephrology* and the *American Journal of Kidney Disease*.

The first book about chelation, called *Metal-Binding in Medicine*, was published in 1960 and included papers that had been presented at two medical symposia. Sadly, lead editor Dr. Martin Seven was killed in a car wreck the following year. As a staunch proponent of chelation therapy with ties to the National Institutes of Health, Seven's untimely death was a huge setback to the acceptance and growth of treatment.

Still, others pressed on. And in 1973, the American Institute of Medical Preventics was formed to promote chelation, as well as train and certify practitioners. The organization later changed its name to the American College for Advancement of Medicine (ACAM) and remains chelation's most prominent training resource and institutional champion.

Meanwhile, several studies were performed with almost uniformly positive results, but they were primarily observational with a limited number of participants, and thus were summarily dismissed by chelation critics. One example is *EDTA Chelation Therapy in the Treatment of Arteriosclerosis and Atherosclerotic Conditions*, a clinical study by integrative physician Dr. Jonathan Collin. Between 1975 and 1981, twenty-six patients with "significant" cardiovascular disease received twenty or more treatments of infused EDTA. Plethysmography, a non-invasive test that can measure plaque buildup in blood vessels, revealed that all twenty-six patients had at least a 20 percent improvement with zero incidences of damage to the kidneys or any other organ.

Doctors Ray Evers and Carlos Lamar amassed volumes of anecdotal evidence that EDTA chelation improved circulation, in some cases saving gangrenous limbs of diabetics suffering from peripheral artery disease. Evers was eventually sued by the FDA for using chelation drugs—which had been FDA-approved only for heavy-metal detoxification—to treat cardiovascular conditions. In 1981, he won a landmark legal case, setting a precedent that allowed doctors to use any FDA-approved drug "off-label" at their own discretion, a common practice today.

In the late 1980s, Walter Reed Army Hospital embarked on a randomized clinical trial of EDTA chelation therapy. But it was interrupted by the Gulf War, which drew away researchers, and was never completed. A handful of randomized, double-blind clinical studies have also been performed, suggesting that EDTA chelation offered no benefits over placebo groups. Two oft-cited trials were published in German journals. The first involved forty-five patients with intermittent claudication, a vascular condition that causes leg pain when walking. In this case, the placebo was the blood-thinning agent bencyclan. Both groups showed similar improvement in symptoms, which researchers explained as "the placebo effect." The second study involved sixteen patients with coronary artery disease. Half had twenty infusions with EDTA, the other half a saline solution. Subjects in both groups noted that they felt better but angiographs and other tests showed no substantial changes in coronary blood flow and a minimal progression of their atherosclerosis. Researchers concluded that chelation had no impact on coronary heart disease.

Dozens of less formal studies were likewise published. One of the most jaw-dropping was performed by Scandinavian doctors Claus Hancke and Knut Flytlie. It involved ninety-two patients who were on waiting lists for either heart bypass operations or limb amputations due to vascular issues. After chelation therapy for an average of six months, the doctors reported that fifty-eight of the sixty-five bypass patients were able to cancel their surgery, and the same held true for twenty-four of the twenty-seven awaiting amputation. A follow-up study years later on forty-seven of the heart patients found that thirty-four of them still hadn't had surgical intervention. In 1992, integrative physician Collin remarked: "If we extrapolate these numbers to the large number of bypass surgeries and amputations performed in the United States, 363,000 of the 407,000 bypass surgeries may have been avoided and 102,000 limbs may have been saved if chelation therapy had been administered to these patients. Furthermore, $8 billion in healthcare costs may have been saved."

Despite a plethora of anecdotal and clinical evidence, there remained a lack of definitive proof in the form of a large, randomized, placebo-controlled, double-blind study that proved chelation therapy really works for anything beyond heavy-metal detoxification. That shortcoming fueled attacks by the medical establishment, including legal assaults that threatened the licenses and livelihoods of practitioners.

Some of the most vicious attacks against chelation were carried out by a band of medical doctors and others who call themselves "skeptics" but are commonly known as "The Quackbusters." Through Internet websites, media outlets, and legal proceedings, they strive to root out fraudulent medical practices. That's not necessarily a bad thing, as there are plenty of unscrupulous people around who take advantage of the desperate and ill-informed with bogus products and therapies. But the Quackbusters tend to target all kinds of alternative practitioners indiscriminately, often in a dismissive, ridiculing manner.

With chelation therapy saddled by a long-ingrained resistance fueled in part by the media-savvy Quackbusters, only a bona fide gold-standard study could possibly quiet the critics and convince the mainstream medical community to give it some respect. And that brings us back to Dr. Tony Lamas and his Trial to Assess Chelation Therapy. For chelation practitioners, Lamas was a great new hope that this therapy they so strongly believed in would finally gain the wide-scale acceptance they felt it deserved.

WHO ARE THE QUACKBUSTERS?

"The Quackbusters" is the informal name for a group of medical doctors and others who basically believe that anything outside of pharmaceutical drugs and surgery is medical heresy. That includes acupuncture, aromatherapy, chiropractic, reflexology, homeopathy, massage therapy, bio-identical hormone replacement, and many others. This also covers disciplines that have gained such widespread acceptance that even tight-fisted insurance companies have had to admit they are medically viable and thus eligible for coverage.

The first prominent Quackbuster was Dr. Morris Fishbein, who sternly ruled the American Medical Association (AMA) for decades and assailed all forms of non-allopathic medicine. Ironically, his efforts were largely financed by the tobacco industry, which paid large sums to advertise in the *Journal of the American Medical Association (JAMA)* with slogans such as L&M cigarettes' "Just what the doctor ordered" or "For digestion's sake, smoke Camels." Fishbein, also known in some circles as the Medical Mussolini, was an MD who never practiced medicine. Until his abrupt ouster from the AMA in 1950, he proved to be a master at propaganda and targeted many alternative practitioners.

Fishbein's legacy lives on in a modern-day set of Quackbusters, who use similar tactics to rip the lid off of what they call "pseudoscience," or basically any medical therapy that drifts outside the lines of drugs and procedures. They operate dozens of websites, including the *National Council Against Health Fraud*, *Science-Based Medicine*, and *Quackwatch*, which reach millions of readers. Some of the Quackbusters have been paid to serve as expert witnesses in trials against alternative medicine practitioners and products. Among those that the Quackbusters have branded "quacks" include the late two-time Nobel laureate Linus Pauling, Dr. Deepak Chopra, Dr. Andrew Weil, and Dr. Mehmet Oz.

One of the Quackbuster ringleaders is Dr. Stephen Barrett, a retired psychiatrist who never passed the tests required to become board-certified. Despite this, he bills himself as a medical and legal expert, even though his only formal legal education consists of a correspondence course from LaSalle University with "one and a half years completed" (according to his curriculum vitae). Like Fishbein, Barrett is masterful at media manipulation. He founded Quackwatch in 1996.

Another luminary following in Fishbein's unseemly footsteps is Dr. Steven Novella, a neurologist who actually *is* board-certified. He founded and regularly blogs on the website Science-Based Medicine, criticizing all forms of alternative disciplines. More concerning though, in 2018 he penned a piece supporting Monsanto (now owned by Bayer) after a jury awarded $289 million to school groundskeeper Dewayne Johnson, who claimed he developed non-Hodgkin's lymphoma due to exposure to the company's flagship product, Roundup. Novella contended there is no reputable science-based link between Roundup's active ingredient glyphosate and lymphoma, or any other cancer. That flies in the face of the World Health Organization's 2015 declaration that glyphosate is a "probable carcinogen." The herbicide is now restricted or banned throughout much of Europe and several other countries due to health concerns, and 13,000 other lymphoma-stricken Roundup users have filed lawsuits against Monsanto/Bayer.

Barrett and Novella are typical of the current band of Quackbusters, who continue Fishbein's disdain of any practice outside allopathic medicine. To their credit, they will occasionally criticize Big Pharma and the AMA for a faux pas or two. And they don't advertise cigarettes.

CHAPTER 5

The Dangers of Heavy Metals and Other Environmentally Acquired Toxins

In the story of chelation, heavy metals are the villains. They insidiously sneak into your body and, like unwelcome house-guests, refuse to leave for years, even decades. They plop down in tissue cells, make a mess of things and certainly don't clean up after themselves. Occasionally, they'll move and settle some-where else—for example migrating from bone to brain tissue. Eventually, they disrupt the function of the cells they inhabit, contributing to degenerative diseases.

The main culprits are lead, mercury, and cadmium, with arsenic, aluminum, and others also in the mix. All of the worst offenders are naturally occurring elements in the earth's soil, but not the human body.

Since the Industrial Revolution began in the eighteenth cen-tury, these heavy metals and other toxic compounds have been increasingly belched into the air and dumped into the water by factories, and a lot of it has eventually wound up back in the soil, but at much higher concentrations. The burning of fossil fuels—whether by powering your car or home—contributes mightily to the contamination, and humans cavalierly rub heavy metals into our sponge-like skin via cosmetics and other personal care products. Many of us have had our teeth filled with a mercury-based alloy. We even suck heavy metals directly into our lungs through cigarette smoke, both actively and passively. Pesticides and some fertilizers contain heavy metals, which adds to their concentration in the soil, and thereby the food chain, so we are constantly ingesting them.

The ways we are exposed to toxic heavy metals goes on and on, and their saturation levels in the environment continue to climb as the planet becomes ever more industrialized. So, if you breathe, eat, drink, and bathe, you are continually adding to your heavy-metal burden.

There is much debate about how much heavy metals affect health. These elements, which are at least five times as dense as water, bind tighter than the essential minerals our bodies need, thus displacing the good things and impairing the functions of cells. They also generate a lot of oxidative stress, causing inflammation and depleting antioxidant reserves. So, in theory, heavy metals could affect any part of your body, either directly or indirectly.

A peer-reviewed manuscript published in the journal *Molecular, Clinical and Environmental Toxicology* states that heavy metals "are systemic toxicants known to induce adverse health effects in humans, including cardiovascular diseases, developmental abnormalities, neurologic and neurobehavioral disorders, diabetes, hearing loss, hematologic and immunologic disorders, and various types of cancer."

Everyone seems to concur that high levels of toxicity—such as in people who work in smelting plants or drink water supplied via corroding lead pipes—are systemically damaging. But not everyone agrees that trace levels of these elements, which slowly accumulate in our tissues over time, have any impact on our health.

Dr. Steven Nissen, Chief Academic Officer of the Cleveland Clinic's Heart and Vascular Institute in Ohio and a staunch chelation critic, says there's simply no scientific proof.

"The idea that we're all contaminated with heavy metals is part of this quack approach in promoting an agenda," Nissen charges. "It's not an accepted finding by the medical community. We have no national guidelines on measuring these things. There's no medical standard. Sure, there's lots of things in the environment, but is it a pathological problem? Cause-and-effect needs to be proven scientifically, and you don't find good quality scientific material to support this."

In fact, there is quite a bit of scientific literature linking detrimental health effects to heavy metals, even at blood levels low enough to be considered acceptable. And the argument could be made that a lack of scientific evidence still wouldn't mean that the problem doesn't exist.

"I don't know how anybody can argue that metals like lead, mercury, and cadmium, which have no role in the human body and are known to be toxic, should remain in the human body," says Dr. Lamas. "It's a mystery to me why we in conventional medicine continue to deny that environmentally acquired toxins are causal agents for a lot of human disease. In cardiology, in particular, we are remarkably thick-headed about this."

And Dr. Tammy Born, whose clinic participated in Lamas' initial TACT study, says she's seeing sicker patients now than she's ever seen in thirty-plus years of practice, and they're getting sick at a younger age.

"We're overloading our bodies not only with heavy metals but also with pesticides, herbicides, hormones, chemicals, antibiotics, and other things that all lower our threshold for disease," she explains. "Nobody's done a study to show what chronic, low-level metal exposure does in a year, or ten years, or fifty years, but we do know we now have a country full of people with cancer, Alzheimer's and heart disease, and maybe this low-grade exposure to toxins is keeping our bodies from working well. Why not at least get the heavy metals out of there with EDTA, which is one of the safest drugs in the world?"

Lamas compares chelation therapy for heavy-metal contamination to a window that hasn't been cleaned for decades.

"You can't see out of it, but if you clean it once, you'll be able to see out of it for years," he says. "It's the same with getting these heavy metals out of your body."

With that in mind, the following is a look at "America's Least Wanted" heavy metals in the body.

Lead

Lead is a high-density metal that is abundant, easily extracted from ores, pliable, resistant to oxidation (rust), and cheap, which made it seemingly great for use in construction, plumbing, bullets, solders, paints, car batteries, as an alloy, and to boost octane in gasoline, among many other things.

On the downside, lead is extremely toxic to human beings and other animals, even in relatively minute amounts. The element (Pb in the Periodic Table) was identified as far back as prehistoric times. The ancient Egyptians used lead in cosmetics. The ancient Chinese used it for contraception. And it was so widely used by the Romans, most notably in their aqueducts, some historians cite it as a contributing factor in the fall of the Roman Empire.

Lead hit its peak usage during the early days of the Industrial Revolution before its extreme toxicity was fully realized. Since the latter half of the twentieth century, efforts have been made to reduce our exposure to the toxin, including the removal of lead from paint and gasoline. But it persists, especially in older buildings—and in our bodies. Lead only stays in the bloodstream for about three months.

About 90 percent of what we absorb during that timeframe settles in bones and teeth, where it can stay for one to several decades, depending on the rate of bone tissue turnover. Children absorb lead up to eight times more efficiently than adults, which is why they are more affected by lead toxicity. Thirty-five years ago, lead levels of 30 micrograms per deciliter (μg/dl) were considered acceptable, but that threshold has been lowered repeatedly through the years.

A 2012 meta-analysis on the health effects of low-level lead exposure performed by the U.S. government's National Toxicology Program found "sufficient" evidence that lead levels below just 5 μg were "associated with adverse health effects in both children and adults." The report considered levels below both 5 μg and 10 μg and, in children, linked them with behavioral problems, decreased cognitive performance, decreased IQ, delayed puberty, decreased growth, and increased susceptibility to allergens.

In adults, links were made to decreased kidney function, high blood pressure, deaths due to cardiovascular issues, hearing loss, cognitive decline, and amyotrophic lateral sclerosis (ALS), a.k.a., Lou Gehrig's disease. Links were also made to low sperm counts in men and, in women, higher rates of miscarriages and premature births, as well as reduced fetal growth of their babies.

Among other things, lead is known to interfere with the ability of the immune system's T-cells to fight cancer, reduce oxygen absorption by degrading hemoglobin, and disrupt calcium metabolism in a way that promotes hardening of the arteries.

"Lead is all around us in relatively low levels, and all of us have some lead burden," says Lamas. "Skeletons of people before the Industrial Revolution have a hundred times less lead in their bones than we do. So, the expectation that having this much lead in our bodies is completely harmless, when we know lead to be a cellular poison, seems nutty to me."

Mercury

Mercury is what made the Mad Hatter mad. The heavy metal commonly found in thermometers, fluorescent bulbs, and tooth fillings was once used by hat-makers in producing felt from animal fur. Inhaling mercury vapors during that process caused erethrism, a neurological disorder informally called "mad hatter's syndrome." That's the origin of Lewis Carrol's "Mad" Hatter character in *Alice's Adventures in Wonderland*. Whereas Carrol's Hatter was comical with his nonsensical ravings and riddles, mercury toxicity is no laughing matter.

Mercury is also not as effectively removed from the body with EDTA, the most commonly used chelating agent, as you'll see when we go into more detail about chelators in the next chapter.

Over the past century, there has been a 3,000 percent increase in environmental mercury levels. Much of it has come from coal-burning industrial plants, as well as factories that use mercury to produce polyvinyl chloride (PVC) and other products. Even though mercury emission levels have been cut by nearly half in the past decade, the element (Hg) persists in the environment. In its liquid metallic form, mercury is relatively inactive. But it vaporizes continuously, and the vapor is extremely toxic.

Besides inhaling mercury vapor from broken thermometers and fluorescent lightbulbs, as well as from environmental sources, many of us are also exposed through our amalgam tooth fillings, an alloy that is 50 percent mercury. Chewing, grinding, brushing, and corrosion is estimated to expose us to between 3 and 17 µg per day. Like other heavy metals, mercury displaces essential metals—such as zinc, cobalt, and nickel—that are needed for enzymatic reactions, causing dysfunction.

"About 80 percent of the mercury vapor you inhale gets absorbed into the body," explains Anne Summers, Ph.D., a professor of microbiology at the University of Georgia. "From the lungs, mercury goes into the bloodstream and runs into (the enzyme) catalase, which converts the uncharged vapor into a positively charged ion that reacts strongly with many biomolecules. Most of the time that's going to be a protein, and the protein is not going to be very happy about that. In fact, it's going to lose function."

We are also exposed to an organic form of the metal called methylmercury through our diet, mostly by eating fish. Large ocean fish, such as tuna, shark, and swordfish, have the highest levels of contamination.

There is much controversy over the health effects of thimerosal, another form of organic mercury. Thimerosal has been used as a preservative in vaccines, an ingredient that some scientists believe contributes to autism and other neurological conditions, even though the CDC has not found a link.

But even without vaccines, we typically carry some amount of mercury in our bodies from environmental and medical exposure, and like lead, there is no safe level. It not only affects virtually all aspects of metabolic function but is also easily transferred from a pregnant woman to her fetus, interfering with brain development.

"Mercury is the most powerful non-radioactive neurotoxin on the planet," says Dr. Nick Meyer, author of *The Holistic Dental Matrix: How Teeth Control Your Health and Well-Being*. "If you have a mercury filling, it continually off-gases. Some people's bodies can excrete mercury in a fairly efficient manner. But if you don't have the right biochemical machinery to get rid of it, that mercury will do a lot of damage."

In a blog, leading functional physician Dr. Mark Hyman adds: "Mercury is lipophilic, meaning that it concentrates in fatty tissues, especially in the brain, which is made mostly of fat. Neurologic symptoms may include encephalopathy (non-specific brain mal-function), nerve damage, Parkinsonian symptoms, tremor, ataxia (loss of balance), impaired hearing, tunnel vision, dysarthria (slurred speech), headache, fatigue, impaired sexual function, and depression."

On a cellular level, mercury has a huge impact on mitochon-dria, the organelles that power cells.

Microbiology professor Summers studies mercury's impact on bacterial proteins that are also found in humans and says: "One of the largest categories of proteins that were affected by mercury were like those in our mitochondria. These proteins play central roles, so if even one of them gets knocked out, it would put the mitochondrion out of business. And mitochondrial fail-ure leads to all kinds of health problems."

Cadmium

Like other heavy metals, cadmium is used in the production of PVC plastics, paint pigments, pesticides, and fertilizers. It's also released into the environment via the burning of fossil fuels, leak-ing sewage sludge, smelting processes, and cigarette smoke.

It's perhaps best known as one of the elements in nickel–cadmium rechargeable batteries. The batteries, which run in the same familiar sizes as alkaline batteries, have been in common use since the mid-twentieth century. Due to the toxic nature of the cadmium (Cd), these batteries are supposed to be disposed of properly. But a majority of them are carelessly discarded and end up in landfills, and thus the environment at large.

In the past few decades, nickel–cadmium batteries have lost a good bit of market share to lithium–ion versions, but more than a billion a year are still being produced, powering portable electronics, toys, tools, and other products.

Cadmium gets into the body through drinking water and food. It's also in the air, so you breathe it in, more so if that air contains tobacco smoke. Cadmium is more highly soluble in water than other metals, so it is more bioactive.

Once inside the body, it binds with red blood cells and accumulates in organs, especially the liver and kidneys. Cadmium has been linked to bone loss, kidney damage, cardiovascular disease, reproductive issues, and various forms of cancer.

"Cadmium competes with zinc in cells, and zinc has a role in thousands of metabolic functions," says Born. "For example, a liver cell that needs zinc to perform certain detoxification functions can't, because the cadmium has displaced the zinc from the cell. And the cadmium is not going anywhere because its half-life can be as long as forty years."

Arsenic

Ask anyone to name a poison, and "arsenic" is likely to be one of the first ones that come to mind. In fact, arsenic was once known as the "King of Poisons" because it has historically been used for murder, at least until a test to detect it was developed in the 1800s. It was also the poison of choice in the stage play and classic 1944 film *Arsenic and Old Lace*.

In truth, arsenic isn't actually a heavy metal but rather a semi-metallic substance called a metalloid. Still, it shares many properties with heavy metals and the ways they can damage the human body.

Arsenic (As) comes in both inorganic (the most toxic) and organic form. The inorganic variety is most commonly used as a wood preservative, which is one reason why you shouldn't burn "pressure treated" wood in the campfire, unless you are wearing a gas mask.

We even absorb trace amounts by walking barefoot on backyard decks or otherwise coming into contact with treated wood. Organic arsenic is commonly used in pesticides, and various forms of it accumulate in seafood. Unlike the inorganic stuff, the body typically gets rid of it before it does much damage.

Arsenic topped both lead and mercury on the most recent Agency for Toxic Substances and Disease Registry Substance Priority List, which ranks environmental toxins for their potential threat to human health due to exposure from hazardous waste sites. Biologically, arsenic interferes with the body's production of adenosine triphosphate (ATP), which is basically the fuel that powers us.

Much of our low-grade exposure to arsenic comes through groundwater. A 2011 study published in the *International Journal of Environmental Research and Public Health* found that more than 40 million U.S. residents had arsenic levels in their public drinking water that were less than half the U.S. standard but still high enough to increase risk for "a range of diseases including hypertension, diabetes, coronary artery disease, skin melanosis, cancer, and poorer cognition."

In particular, long-term exposure to these "acceptable" levels of arsenic in drinking water affected neuropsychological functioning, and could be an underlying factor in the development of Alzheimer's disease.

Other Metals

Aluminum

Strong and lightweight, aluminum (Al) is the most abundant metal on the planet. While it may be great for airplane fuselages and soda cans, there is no role for aluminum in the human body.

Though we ingest fairly high amounts in food and drugs (especially from antacid medications), only about 1 percent gets into the bloodstream, and most of that is excreted in urine. So, no adverse effects have been identified from this type of exposure. There have been concerns about topical exposure through the workplace, cosmetics, and especially via antiperspirants, which use aluminum to clog sweat glands. You also breathe in the aluminum-laden aerosol mist, providing a beeline to the brain through the olfactory system. Still, most studies have found no link between these types of exposure and chronic disease.

The same goes for aluminum cookware. Some Alzheimer's patients have elevated levels of aluminum, but no definitive link has been found. However, a lot remains unknown, and the consensus of scientists is that there is likely no safe level of aluminum. Ominously, the explosion of Alzheimer's cases parallels the usage curve of aluminum since World War II. More research is needed, but in the meantime, experts suggest taking a precautionary approach and trying to minimize exposure as much as possible.

Iron

An essential trace mineral, iron (Fe) is a component of hemoglobin, a substance in red blood cells that carries oxygen. Deficiencies can cause anemia, which is marked by extreme fatigue but can affect every part of the body. Too much iron is toxic.

Fortunately, our bodies are pretty good at regulating iron levels. Iron overloads mainly affect people with the genetic disorder hemochromatosis.

Chromium

Another essential trace mineral, chromium (Cr) is needed by the body, primarily for glucose metabolism. But the nutritional form (trivalent) is different from the toxic industrial form (hexavalent). The latter is used to produce paint pigments, rubber, cement, and paper and wood preservatives, among other things. Often, it gets into the environment through the leather-tanning process.

It is also contained in cigarette smoke. At this point, no one is sure what chronic low-level exposure to chromium does, though it likely affects enzymatic reactions by displacing essential minerals. Acute exposure is known to be carcinogenic and is especially tough on the lungs, liver, kidneys, and intestinal tract.

The heavy metals covered in this chapter are the usual suspects in human health problems, but there are about three dozen in all that may play a role.

IN THEIR OWN WORDS

When I was nineteen, I started working at a refinery in southeast Texas. I was a pipe-fitter and welder, and I had a lot of chemical and metal exposure. As time went on, I developed a whole plethora of health problems: skin problems, digestive problems, and chronic fatigue that got so bad I had trouble walking from my house to my mom's house, and it was only about twenty yards away. A test showed I had every toxic metal known to man in me and enough mercury to kill a horse. I had the metal removed from my mouth and over a hundred chelation infusions.

Gradually, I got better and am a normal person today. I still chelate monthly and will for the rest of my life. Chelation brought me out of the depths of hell.

Gary R., 61, Beaumont, Texas

CHAPTER 6

What Are Chelators and How Do They Work?

The acceptable levels of heavy metals in our bodies have dropped dramatically through the years, and it's why groups, including the World Health Organization, warn that there are no safe levels of lead, mercury, cadmium, and others of their heavy-metal ilk.

That's why chelation offers a powerful solution. These negatively charged substances have the ability to round up the positively charged Bad Guys (heavy metals) and show them the door, which in this case is mostly through the urethra.

"Chelators have a pocket with an electrical charge, almost like a baseball mitt with a magnet in it," Dr. Lamas explained during a 2019 presentation to a group of vascular specialists. "As with a mitt catching a baseball, the chelator will capture positive ions—for example, toxic metals, such as lead or cadmium—and hold onto them. The metals pass through the body and are excreted in the urine."

Due to their varied chemical structures and bonding capabilities, chelating agents have different affinities for specific metals, which is why some are better for lead, while others may be better for mercury or arsenic, and so on.

Disodium EDTA

As you may recall from our lesson in chelation history, the primary soldier in the battle against heavy metals is disodium ethylenediaminetetraacetic acid (EDTA). It was first used as therapy for heart patients back in the 1950s and remains the go-to drug for chelation practitioners today. It's important to realize that disodium EDTA is always delivered via infusion and can only be prescribed by a medical doctor (MD) or doctor of osteopathy (DO). So, you should avoid being treated with it by a chiropractor or any other practitioner who doesn't have the legal power to prescribe pharmaceutical drugs, as well as a certification in IV chelation. Disodium EDTA has FDA approval only for treating super-high blood calcium levels and one type of heart arrhythmia. However, physicians can prescribe it "off-label," meaning for a different use, based on their belief of what is best for the patient.

Lamas uses disodium EDTA in his TACT studies. He follows a long-established protocol endorsed, taught, and certified by the American College for Advancement in Medicine (ACAM), the International College of Integrative Medicine (ICIM), and the International Board of Clinical Metal Toxicology (IBCMT).

That protocol consists of three grams of disodium EDTA mixed with magnesium, vitamin C, sterile water, and other substances (see the box). It is typically infused at a rate of one gram of EDTA per hour. So, a three-gram dose takes three hours. Infusing it at a faster rate risks kidney damage, because that would expose the delicate, bean-shaped organs to a tsunami of heavy metals, minerals, and other things that can overwhelm them and cause a condition called acute tubular necrosis. Pretty much anything with "necrosis" in its name is bad news, in this case meaning it can kill cells in the kidneys' filtration system.

HOW TO REDUCE HEAVY-METAL EXPOSURE

Although heavy metals are everywhere, there are certain things you can do to limit your exposure to them, including:

- Quit smoking. Tobacco smoke contains some of the worst of the Bad Guys—arsenic, cadmium and lead—as well as many chemical toxins. This is not only unhealthy for you but anyone who inhales your secondhand smoke.
- Replace amalgam tooth fillings with a composite material. Be sure your dentist is trained in how to do this safely, or the vapors released could harm you and even the dental staff.
- Limit consumption of some seafood, particularly large ocean fish such as tuna, shark, and swordfish.
- Install a reverse-osmosis water filter in your house, which will remove all toxins, including heavy metals.
- Inspect older houses for lead paint and other possible heavy-metal sources.
- Wear protective equipment if you have occupational exposure through work, hobbies, or other activities that may put you in increased contact with these substances.
- Be sure to properly dispose of batteries, fluorescent bulbs, and other toxic metal–containing products through programs and facilities designed to keep them from getting into the environment.

Even worse, getting too much EDTA too fast can also cause a sudden drop in blood calcium levels, possibly resulting in abnormal electrical activity in the heart and brain, two organs you definitely don't want to mess with. So low blood calcium levels, called hypocalcemia, can have deadly consequences. Fortunately, none of these bad things happen if the EDTA is infused at the proper rate, which must be pretty idiot-proof considering the hundreds of thousands of infusions performed every year in the U.S. without serious incident.

However, chelation critics will always cite those three tragic cases in the early 2000s, where two children and an adult died as a result of unqualified practitioners who basically overdosed them by injecting the drug too rapidly. In those cases, disodium EDTA was accidentally given instead of calcium disodium EDTA, a variation of the drug (usually called "calcium EDTA"), which has no effect on blood calcium levels and can be infused faster, provided the kidneys can handle the load of metals coming out.

"If you're working with physicians who know what they're doing and follow the protocol, EDTA is safer than Tylenol, by far," declares Lamas. "The dangers have been overblown to the nth degree."

For those interested in a treatment that is statistically safer than a top-selling over-the-counter pain reliever, each infusion under the standard protocol takes three hours. That can be a big chunk of the day, especially for people who are still gainfully employed. But it can actually be done faster without compromising safety or efficacy.

A 1994 analysis of nineteen studies involving 22,765 patients found that 87 percent of them showed improvements in vascular function after having chelation therapy. But in one of the studies, 2,482 patients were infused with just 1.5 grams of EDTA at a time, and they reaped the same benefits. Around the same time, the late

Dr. Grant Born co-directed a study in which thirty patients with peripheral artery disease were given twenty infusions of either 3-gram or 1.5-gram EDTA solutions, and a Doppler ultrasound used to measure plaque reduction in arteries showed that the 1.5-gram group actually averaged better results by a statistically significant margin. Other studies support the findings that a 1.5-gram dose works at least as well as a 3-gram dose.

That's good news to patients, because it cuts the length of the treatment session from three hours to just ninety minutes. Still, it's recommended that patients get no more than three treatments a week with at least twenty-four hours between them.

And people with kidney issues need special attention, which usually involves estimating the glomerular filtration rate (how effectively the kidneys are filtering the blood) by testing levels of creatinine (a waste product the kidneys excrete) to make sure they can tolerate the toxic metals passing through them. In nearly seventy years of chelation therapy for vascular disease, no fatalities have been attributed to it when the protocol is followed.

So, despite the unfortunate incidents in the early 2000s, disodium EDTA infusions will not hurt you if administered properly by a qualified practitioner. Do your research and find a practitioner who has been trained by either the American College for Advancement in Medicine or the International College of Integrative Medicine. Typically, the worst side effect is a burning sensation at the site of the IV needle. In my personal experience having chelation infusions at the Born Clinic, I didn't even feel that.

Among other things, disodium EDTA:

- Inhibits the destructive peroxidation process of fat molecules in cells, thus preserving the internal membranes needed to maintain cellular health.

- Protects mitochondria—the power generators of cells—from oxidative damage that can impair the process of turning nutrients into energy.
- Limits the coagulating capability of platelets to reduce the risk of potentially catastrophic clots forming inside of blood vessels.
- Improves bone structure by lowering blood calcium levels, which stimulates the release of parathormone, a hormone that enhances dissolution of metastatic calcium in blood vessels and joints, and relocation of that calcium in bone cells.

Because EDTA removes some essential minerals along with the toxic metals, patients are given supplements to bolster those levels. Studies show that the chelation of essential minerals such as zinc and manganese is minimal, much less than the recommended daily allowance, and can easily be replaced. So, the net loss is nothing but Bad Guys.

Calcium EDTA

Calcium EDTA is another form of the substance used in chelation therapy. This is the version approved by the FDA for acute heavy-metal toxicity, and is most commonly prescribed for lead poisoning. In chelation therapy, it is often employed when first evaluating a patient, during the so-called "challenge test." Remember that heavy metals don't typically circulate in the bloodstream longer than a few weeks, but rather settle in tissue.

So, unless you have a lot of recent or constant exposure, blood and urine levels of toxic metals will remain low, even if your tissues are loaded with them. The calcium EDTA will extract some metals from tissue, and they will show up in the urine.

The procedure goes something like this: You collect a sample of urine for a baseline measure before a dose of calcium EDTA is injected into your bloodstream. Then you collect your urine over the course of six hours or more. Both samples are sent to a lab, and the post-chelation batch is likely to contain much higher levels of heavy metals than the pre-chelation sample. Lamas says the average during his first TACT study was nearly a 4,000 percent increase in urinary lead and 700 percent increase in cadmium.

Still, those numbers may be deceptive because even 4,000 percent of a miniscule amount may not add up to much. In truth, it is very difficult to determine heavy-metal toxicity, and even more difficult to assess how much it may be affecting an individual's health. Due to genetic factors, as well as exposure to other toxins, and lifestyle and additional variables, some people can tolerate higher levels than others without their health being measurably impacted. But the bottom line is that these metals have no purpose in human physiology and can't be doing us any good. Presumably, the less of them you have, the better.

Like its brother disodium EDTA, the calcium version doesn't stay in the body very long. It latches on to heavy metals and a smattering of minerals, then splits, usually within twenty-four hours.

By the way, our bodies are already quite familiar with calcium EDTA, because it is a very common FDA-approved food additive, used in things like mayonnaise, salad dressings, pickled vegetables, canned legumes, and carbonated soft drinks. Its chelating properties help to preserve the food's flavor, texture, and color, as well as its shelf life. It is also used to neutralize the chemically active heavy metals used in cosmetics, detergents, and a host of other personal care and household products.

The biggest physiological difference between the two commonly used EDTAs is that the calcium version does not bind with calcium in the bloodstream. That makes it even more idiot-proof than disodium EDTA, and it's why it's the type normally used for acute heavy-metal toxicity, such as for the children who got lead poisoning from drinking the tainted water in Flint, Michigan.

While safer to inject quickly, the lack of calcium-binding properties may make it a less-efficient therapy for atherosclerosis because it won't affect calcium deposits in blood vessels as much or reduce the potentially dangerous blood clotting factors of platelets. However, by lightening the load of toxic metals, it still is likely to clear arteries and improve circulation in various other ways.

Calcium EDTA is also available in oral form, but its absorption rate is estimated to be a paltry 5 percent compared with nearly 100 percent of the infused variety. Oral EDTA is also considered a supplement and not a medication, so it doesn't require a prescription or undergo the same scrutiny as the intravenous drug.

Some of the products that anyone can buy on the Internet are not formulated carefully and may even have metal contaminants, which could defeat the purpose of the treatment. That said, for people who can't spend the money or time on infused EDTA, a good quality oral version may help. It certainly seems to have worked for Angie Divoso.

During a regular checkup a few years ago, her primary physician, West Bloomfield, Michigan–based Dr. David Brownstein, heard a "whooshing sound" in one of her carotid arteries through his stethoscope and suggested she see a vascular specialist.

"I got an ultrasound and it showed I had 90 percent blockage in that carotid and 30 percent blockage in the other," recalls the now 78-year-old semi-retired hairdresser. "The vascular doctor told me I needed surgery or I could have a stroke.

"It was a shock to me, and I started putting names on my jewelry for my kids because I thought I might die. But the idea of surgery scared me, so I went back to Dr. Brownstein and he said we could try chelation."

Brownstein, one of the country's top holistic medicine practitioners and author of the *Natural Way to Health* newsletter, put Angie on oral calcium EDTA. She says she took one capsule at bedtime for about five months.

"At that point, Dr. Brownstein could no longer hear that rushing sound in my neck," says Angie. "And when the vascular doctor gave me an ultrasound, he said I had no blockage in either of my carotids. He was surprised and at a loss to explain it. I didn't tell him about the chelation because a lot of doctors think you're crazy to do it. I just told him it must be an intervention from God above. He said he wanted to see me in six months, but I never went back."

Another option that seems to be gaining in popularity is a calcium EDTA suppository. One study using lab rats shows that it has a respectable 36 percent absorption rate and actually stays in the body hours longer than the infused version.

"I do a lot more suppositories and oral EDTA chelation than intravenous," says integrative physician Dr. Robert Rowen. "I stress methods that people can do at home. The suppositories take about three times as long to work as the infusions, but they get the job done with more convenience and at a lower cost."

Still, most chelation practitioners will tell you if you have heart disease, peripheral artery disease, or some other critical problem, your best bet is disodium EDTA infusions, along with some of the other chelators listed next.

DMPS and DMSA

As mentioned earlier, while EDTA is a very effective chelator for lead and cadmium, it is not an effective chelator for mercury, which we mostly get from amalgam tooth fillings, eating seafood, and breathing in an atmosphere containing burnt fossil fuel byproducts. Dimercapto propanesulfonic acid (DMPS) and dimercaptosuccinic acid (DMSA) may be preferable to, or used in addition to, EDTA in some cases. Infused DMPS (also called unithiol) is commonly used in Russia and Europe for heavy-metal toxicity, but it hasn't been approved for treatment of anything in the U.S. However, it remains on the FDA's "bulk compounding list," meaning it can be legally used when produced by compounding pharmacies. It's also available in an oral version. Along with mercury, it binds tightly with zinc and copper, two essential trace minerals. So, supplements for them are highly recommended.

"DMPS as an injectable has an 18 percent chance of significant side effects, but the oral version is actually incredibly safe and effective," says leading integrative family physician Dr. John Parks Trowbridge. "The problem is that it's readily available all over the world, but not in the United States. The FDA is exceptionally good at decreasing access to items that work very well and have been putting the squeeze on chelators, making them hard to get and more expensive. It's very frustrating."

DMSA (also called succimer) is a modified version of British anti-lewisite (BAL), a chelating agent developed as an antidote to weaponized lewisite poison used during World War II. But it also can chelate lead, mercury, arsenic, and other heavy metals. DMSA has similar capabilities to BAL but fewer harmful side effects, so it has replaced BAL. DMSA is FDA-approved for the treatment of lead poisoning in children.

And like DMPS, it also has a strong affinity for methylmercury (the kind you get from eating seafood). It's only used orally, and triggers the release of the metal from soft tissue. DMSA is often utilized in addition to EDTA or DMPS infusions. Some practitioners use it for the challenge test instead of the injected calcium EDTA.

Mercury Levels in Seafood

High	Low
Bluefish	Artic Cod
Crab (Blue)	Anchovies
Grouper	Butterfish
Mackerel (King, Spanish, Gulf)	Catfish
Marlin	Clam
Orange Roughy	Crab (Domestic)
Salmon (Farmed, Atlantic)	Crawfish
Seabass (Chilean)	Croaker (Atlantic)
Shark	Flounder
Swordfish	Haddock (Atlantic)
Tilefish	Hake
Tuna (Ahi, Yellowfin, Bigeye, Blue, Canned Albacore)	Herring
Medium:	Mackerl (North Atlantic, Chub)
Bass (Striped)	Mullet
Carp	Oyster
Cod (Alaskan)	Perch (Ocean)
Croaker (White Pacific)	Plaice
Halibut (Atlantic, Pacific)	Pollock
Lobster	Salmon (Canned, Fresh, Wild)
Mahi Mahi	Sardine
Monkfish	Scallop
Perch (Freshwater)	Shad
Sablefish	Squid
Skate	Talapia
Snapper	Trout
Tuna (Canned Chunk Light, Skipjack)	Whitefish
Sea Trout	Whiting

"I use oral DMSA in conjunction with IV EDTA, because you're not going to chelate all of the mercury out of anybody using EDTA alone," says Dr. Joe Hickey, a prominent integrative internist. "Using DMSA with the infusion and for a couple of days afterward will also help prevent any redistribution of lead and other heavy metals after they are released from the bone."

Because DMSA doesn't permeate cell membranes, it needs help from glutathione, a super-antioxidant that our own bodies produce naturally. Glutathione pushes metals out of cells for the DMSA to haul off, kind of like setting your trash by the side of the road for the garbage truck to take away. Because supplies of glutathione are limited, DMSA is taken in cycles—for example, three days straight, then five to eleven days off of it. That gives the body time to regenerate its glutathione supply.

Alpha-Lipoic Acid (ALA)

Our bodies produce ALA, a powerful antioxidant and chelator that can cross cell membranes as well as the blood–brain barrier, a special safeguard that protects our most precious organ. That's important because lead and mercury, in particular, like to hunker down in brain tissue, where they can contribute to a whole spectrum of cognitive problems. ALA not only chelates heavy metals but also protects cell membranes from their oxidizing effects.

ALA is found to a small degree in foods, including spinach, broccoli, Brussels sprouts, peas, and organ meats. Because our bodies only produce small amounts of it, and it's hard to get a lot of it from our diet, supplementation is often recommended. As an added bonus, ALA boosts the body's production of glutathione which, as we've already noted, is great at extracting metals from tissue but constantly needs to be replenished.

PRACTITIONER PROFILE
DR. JOHN PARKS TROWBRIDGE

Life Celebrating Health, Humble, Texas
Undergraduate: Stanford University,
Biological Sciences, 1970
Medical School: Case Western Reserve
University, 1976
Specialty: Integrative family medicine
Selected Honors and Associations:
- Who's Who Top Doctor in Advanced
  Medicine
- Who's Who Lifetime Achievement
  Award
- Distinguished Lifetime Achievement Award, International
  College of Integrative Medicine
- American College for Advancement in Medicine, Fellow
- Preventive Medicine, Medical Research Institute of Florida
  Institute of Technology, Diplomate, 1985
- Chelation Therapy, Diplomate, 1985
- International College of Integrative Medicine, President
- International Academy of Biological Dentistry and Medicine,
  President
- NeuroCranial Research Institute, President
- National Health Federation, Director
- American College for Advancement in Medicine, Officer and
  Director
- American Board of Clinical Metal Toxicology, Officer and
  Director
- American Preventive Medical Association, Charter Director
- Best-selling author of *The Yeast Syndrome* (Bantam Books)

Website: https://healthchoicesnow.com

Quote: "I tell everybody that chelation does three things.
Number One, it removes toxic metals. Number Two, it
removes toxic metals. And Number Three, it removes toxic
metals. If you keep those three things in mind, you can clearly
understand how chelation benefits health. Toxic metals interfere with normal body metabolism, and that means healing,
repair, normal function . . . everything. If you just get them out
of the way, the body can heal itself."

N-Acetyl Cysteine (NAC)

NAC is not only an effective oral chelator in itself, it also increases levels of the ever-important glutathione. Side benefits include keeping lung tissue moist through its mucus-thinning effects, protecting the liver from alcohol byproducts and the pain-relieving drug acetaminophen, and increasing red blood cell production. Diabetics should consult their doctors about taking it due to its potential to affect insulin production.

D-Penicillamine

This derivative of penicillin is most commonly used for an overload of copper in the very few people who suffer from Wilson's disease. Sometimes, it serves as an adjunctive treatment for lead and arsenic poisoning. It's also used to treat some rheumatoid arthritis patients. Because it has a different chemical composition than penicillin, people who are allergic to the antibacterial drug are not at higher risk for an allergy to d-penicillamine.

"I like d-penicillamine, but it's very hard to get these days and much more expensive than it used to be," grouses Trowbridge.

Deferoxamine (DFO)

Most widely used as an iron chelator, DFO also binds with copper and aluminum, which all have a triple-plus charge. Trowbridge uses it in injectable form, typically with every fifth EDTA infusion, depending on the patient's needs.

While we need some iron, elevated levels are tough on blood vessels. Iron affects all of the cell types—endothelial, macrophages, smooth muscle, and platelets—that participate in the artery-clogging process. It is seen as a risk factor for heart disease, along with things like diabetes, hypertension, obesity, smoking, and family history.

"We call DFO the 'extra chelator,'" says Trowbridge. "It looks for things like iron and copper, which are physiological metals but toxic when they are in the wrong places. The deferoxamine is very expensive. Only one company in the world makes it, and they've said they were going to stop. So we don't know how long it will be available."

CHELATION INFUSION RECIPE

Here are the ingredients of the infusions used in the TACT studies, their roles explained by Dr. John Parks Trowbridge, Diplomate of the American Board of Chelation Therapy (1985).

3 grams disodium EDTA: An FDA-approved "chelator," disodium EDTA is a chemical compound that attaches to various metals (such as lead, cadmium, and others) so they are removed harmlessly through the urine.

7 grams ascorbate: A form of vitamin C that amplifies the effects of many compounds in the body. It restores more normal structures and functions in many systems, and likely increases the results from EDTA chelation.

2 grams magnesium chloride: Makes the disodium EDTA infusion much more comfortable. It also efficiently adds to body stores of this essential mineral that's required in more than 300 enzyme functions.

100 milligrams procaine hydrochloride: Also makes infusion more comfortable and acts as a membrane stabilizer, helping to restore better health to a variety of cells.

2,500 units heparin: A "touch" of anti-coagulant that allows blood to flow more readily into the tiniest blood vessels (arterioles and capillaries), reaching deeper into body tissues.

2 milliequivalents potassium chloride: This essential body mineral assists EDTA in restoring a more normal chemical balance in body cells.

840 milligrams sodium bicarbonate: A natural "buffer" that changes the acidity/alkalinity of the IV solution to make it more easily tolerated by the blood vessels.

250 milligrams pantothenic acid: An essential B5 vitamin that participates in many enzyme reactions in most body cells and protects them from damage by chemicals and other stressors.

100 milligrams thiamine: An essential B1 vitamin that participates in many enzyme reactions and enhances the removal of lead when combined with EDTA.

100 milligrams pyridoxine: An essential B6 vitamin that participates in many enzyme reactions and reduces some possible side effects found with EDTA administration.

Sterile water to top off 500 milliliters of solution: A dilution of IV constituents that provides a comfortable and tolerable "osmolality" (concentration of particles in solution), so that the infusion is not irritating to the vein lining.

Selenium

This trace mineral has a high binding affinity with mercury. It is yet another vital substance in the production of glutathione.

In China, 103 workers exposed to mercury were given either 100 micrograms of selenium a day or a placebo. The active group (selenium takers) showed more mercury excretion and a reduction of inflammation and oxidative stress markers than the placebo group. Selenium supplements are available, but Brazil nuts are loaded with it. Eating just two or three of them a day will give you all the selenium you need. The nuts also have protein, healthy fats, fiber, and a host of other essential trace minerals.

Silicon and Zeolites

The mineral silicon, as well as zeolite compounds, possess a crystalline structure that encourages binding with heavy metals, especially aluminum. As we've noted before, Alzheimer's disease patients tend to have elevated levels of aluminum. Clinical studies suggest that these compounds support cognitive function and may potentially reduce the risk of Alzheimer's disease.

Vitamin C

What isn't this vitamin good for? A great antioxidant, vitamin C protects cells against heavy metals and reduces the body's absorption of them. Studies show the higher the blood levels of vitamin C, the lower the levels of lead. While oral supplements may help, infusions of Vitamin C are more effective. In fact, seven grams of it are included in the standard disodium EDTA solution.

Select Foods

Some foods contain chelating compounds or otherwise support the body's ability to rid itself of heavy metals. They include cilantro, garlic, chlorella, spirulina, dulse (brown seaweed), green tea, and curry. Foods to avoid include some seafood (especially farmed fish and fish high on the food chain), brown rice (high arsenic levels), produce that is not organically grown, and unfiltered water.

"While foods can help and selections are important, they are not sufficient to reduce the burden of toxic metals in people," notes Trowbridge.

Fiber, Water, and Probiotics

No matter how you wrest heavy metals from tissue, some of it is going to end up in your digestive tract. And if it just sits there because you are constipated or dehydrated, it could be reabsorbed. So, do yourself a favor and eat some high-fiber foods (fruit, vegetables, legumes, and whole grains), drink plenty of purified water, and top it all off with some microbiome-boosting probiotics.

CHAPTER 7

Heavy Metals
and Heart Disease

Dr. John Parks Trowbridge likes to tell this joke to illustrate the shortcomings of conventional medicine:

> A guy who has had too many drinks is crawling around on all fours on a corner by a streetlight when a fella comes along and asks him what he's doing.
> "Why, I'm ... I'm looking for my car keys."
> "Do you remember where you last had them?"
> "Yeah, shh ... shure," he slurs. "Over there, across the street."
> "Then why are you looking here?"
> "Because the light's sooo much better over here."

Trowbridge lets loose a hearty laugh. "That's indeed what most doctors do," he says.

The point is that even though there is really little to no hope in finding lasting cures to disease through the typical conventional therapies—drugs and procedures—doctors persist in using them because that is what they are trained to do, and it is in their comfort zone. They tend to be wary, if not downright hostile, toward anything that lies outside of that well-lit arena.

Trowbridge ought to know. He was once among their numbers. He was a conventional family doctor in 1981 when his father, who had previously needed an aortic replacement, said his chiropractor recommended chelation.

"I told my dad I didn't want him to do it because if it was any good, I would have heard about it," he recalls. "I thought it might even be quackery."

But the following year, while visiting his ailing mother in San Francisco, he met an alternative practitioner who used chelation and was surprised that Trowbridge hadn't heard much about it.

"He took me into the infusion room at his office and told me, 'Here's my nurse. Here's my charts. Here's my patients. Have a good day,'" says Trowbridge. "Well, that was a mind-blowing experience. I could talk to the nurse, look at the charts, and talk to the patients in detail. I was absolutely persuaded that chelation was an incredible tool and started reading everything I could about it. I got trained in the procedure, then traveled to the top ten chelation clinics in the country and stole all of their best ideas. I began using chelation in my practice on June 1, 1983."

Believing that chelation was "a better mousetrap," Trowbridge tried to spread the word by writing an article about it for the local newspaper. That sparked a rebuttal by doctors at the hospital where he was affiliated, and they soon launched a drive to revoke his hospital privileges, which could have resulted in the summary loss of his medical license. An eight-year legal battle ensued, with Trowbridge finally prevailing and being cleared of all challenges to his position on the hospital staff.

"Two weeks after I was reinstated, I resigned," he says. "I've continued practicing in my office ever since, and I consider chelation to be the crown jewel of what we do here."

He's still going strong at age seventy-two. Regarded as one of the top integrative doctors in the country, Trowbridge is a best-selling author and practices in Humble, Texas, treating patients who affectionately call him Dr. T.

"I told Dr. T, if more people actually knew what happens in the rooms of his office, there would be a line down the hall, down the stairs, out the building, and around the corner," says 80-year-old retired schoolteacher Helen Higdon, who gets monthly chelation infusions as a preventive measure. "He's an amazing man who really cares about his patients."

Heavy Metals and Heart Disease

While chelation is just one tool in Dr. T's toolbox of therapies, it is a key one. He and other practitioners will tell you that chelation doesn't just mask symptoms like most drugs, but rather treats a physiologically disruptive problem at its source. By reducing the load of toxic metals in the body, chelation battles any disease that is affected by cellular function—which is pretty much every chronic disease.

Another integrative physician, Dr. David Brownstein, says: "In testing thousands of people, our experience has been that nearly 100 percent of them are toxic from heavy metals. The cells are sick from these metals, and they need to be cleaned out to function normally."

Without being burdened by lead, mercury, cadmium, and the other Bad Guys in our story, cells are more efficient doing the things they were designed to do, such as replicate accurately, create energy, protect and repair themselves, communicate with each other, and dispose of their own waste. Breakdowns in one or more of these areas can cause dysfunction, which eventually leads to disease, particularly the age-related varieties such as cancer, type 2 diabetes, dementia, arthritis, and others.

But chelation could have the biggest impact on public health by combating heart disease, which has reigned as the undisputed national champ of killing Americans since knocking pneumonia from that perch in the 1920s. Heart disease is now responsible for one in four deaths in this country. It also costs about $200 billion a year in medical expenses, medications, and lost productivity, not to mention exacting an enormous emotional toll on patients and their loved ones.

The most common cause of heart disease, and other cardiovascular conditions, is arteriosclerosis, or "hardening" of the arteries, and the resulting atherosclerosis, the narrowing of arteries due to plaque buildup. This can lead to ischemia, which are blockages in arteries that damage tissue by stopping blood flow to it.

As we age, we tend to accumulate deposits of plaque inside of blood vessels, which clog up the plumbing. Plaque not only constricts blood flow and raises pressure, it can also rupture, producing blood clots that cause myocardial infarction (heart attack), stroke, lung embolism, and some other things that are sure to ruin your day.

Bypass, Stents, and Drugs

One way to deal with clogged-up cardiac arteries is to perform coronary artery bypass graft surgery (CABG). Argentine surgeon Dr. Rene Favaloro performed the first successful one on a human at the Cleveland Clinic in 1967. While it's widely documented that the patient was a 51-year-old woman, it's not so easy to find out anything else about her, like how long she lived. In any case, it must have worked pretty well seeing how CABG became the go-to treatment for people with really bad angina or blockages in major cardiac arteries.

Besides being relatively risky surgery, CABG—the most widely practiced version of graft bypass surgery—seems downright barbaric. Typically, a surgeon cuts you open from just below your Adam's apple to just above your navel. Then, your breastbone is sawed through and peeled back to expose your heart. To do the grafts, your heart is stopped, which means redirecting the blood flow through a cardiopulmonary (heart-lung) bypass machine.

Historically, the "donor" grafts are leg veins you apparently don't really need. One end is sewn into the aorta and the other end is sewn into the occluded coronary artery below the blockage, bypassing it like a detour on the Interstate.

One problem with CABG is that the grafts often fail. A 2011 study at Johns Hopkins estimated that half of all venous grafts went kaput within ten years, in part because veins were not designed to do the work of arteries. And whatever forces—genetic, lifestyle, environmental, or a combination of all three—clogged up the vessels in the first place can eventually clog up the grafts.

Nowadays, some "off-pump" heart bypasses are done without stopping the heart, and cutting-edge robotic surgery performs it through small incisions rather than open-chest, using more suitable mammalian arteries from the chest for the grafts.

Considering the chest is usually cracked open and the heart is stopped, it may come as no surprise that the mortality rate of CABG is relatively high. According to The Society of Thoracic Surgeons, between 1 and 2 percent of CABG patients die during the procedure or within thirty days of it, most often from heart attacks. While that percentage may sound low, it still works out to more than 2,000 people a year. For the vast majority who survive, the complication rate is a more substantial 20 to 30 percent and includes increased risk of stroke, chronic lung or kidney disease, abnormal heart rhythms, and cognitive impairment.

Despite its drawbacks, CABG surgery is firmly established as the standard of care for people with potentially life-threatening blockages or severe chest pain from angina that has failed to respond to other treatments. While surgery may fix the problem, for some heart patients the reprieve is temporary, and many of them will eventually need to have the old grafts reamed out or replaced by new ones.

The number of CABGs being performed has been dropping in recent years due to advances in percutaneous coronary intervention (PCI), a tongue-twisting name for a minimally invasive procedure that opens up clogged or partially clogged arteries. Most commonly, this consists of a balloon angioplasty and stent implantation. A catheter is threaded through a blood vessel—typically in the groin—all the way to the constricted part of the coronary artery. At that point, a balloon in the tip of the catheter is inflated, smooshing the fatty plaque against the wall of the artery and thus opening up the vessel to allow better blood flow. To prevent the fatty plaque from expanding after being compressed, a scaffolding called a stent is implanted to help keep the artery open.

Certainly, a PCI is far less traumatic than undergoing CABG and being cut open like a freshly caught trout. If you're having a heart attack, it can quickly restore blood flow to the area of the heart served by that particular vessel, limiting irreversible tissue damage. Most often it is used to relieve the chest pain caused by angina pectoris, which can be "stable" (pain upon physical exertion or stress) or "unstable" (pain even while at rest). A majority of the stent implantations every year are performed on stable angina patients, and it has a high rate of success in relieving pain.

The downside is that the procedure can damage the blood vessel or cause heart rhythm problems. If scar tissue forms around the stent, another procedure may be needed to clear it out. And because stents promote the formation of blood clots, patients are commonly put on blood-thinning anticoagulant medication for a long time, if not for life. While that may come in handy to prevent blood clots forming around stents, it's not very helpful if you have an accident with a knife or chainsaw or anything else that causes bleeding, because the drugs make the flow much harder to staunch.

There is a lot of controversy raging over whether PCI is the best option for stable angina patients. Two mostly ignored studies from more than a decade ago show that treating the condition with "medical management" (medications and lifestyle adjustments) alone is even more successful than stents in preventing death from all causes, as well as from heart attacks and other cardiac events.

The Occluded Artery Trial (OAT) in 2006 found that opening totally clogged arteries with stents after "uncomplicated" heart attacks actually increased mortality rates slightly when compared to medical management. And the 2007 Clinical Outcomes Utilizing Revascularization and Aggressive Drug Evaluation (COURAGE) study found that stents were no more effective than proper medical management for stable coronary artery disease.

In combining their study with others, totaling 5,000 patients, the COURAGE researchers concluded that "PCI has no effect in reducing major cardiovascular events." A 2012 editorial in *JAMA* cited COURAGE and other studies in blasting stent implantation on stable heart disease patients as "an expensive placebo" for pain relief. The editorial even questioned whether it was time for the practitioners who vigorously defended stents to "abandon ship."

Oddly enough, physicians who claim to be science-based paid little heed to those studies and the *JAMA* editorial. It may be harder for them to ignore a more recent trial that sent shockwaves through the cardiology community when it was presented at the American Heart Association Scientific Sessions in November 2019. The $100 million International Study of Comparative Health Effectiveness with Medical and Invasive Approaches (ISCHEMIA) found no evidence that patients with moderate to severe heart disease who underwent invasive PCI or CABG procedures experienced reduced rates of major cardiac events—such as death and heart attacks—than those treated with drugs and lifestyle changes alone.

ISCHEMIA did show that interventions reduced chest pain and thus improved quality of life for some patients. But the truth of the matter is that a majority of the procedures are performed on people with no or infrequent symptoms.

"For people without symptoms, who've either never had symptoms or who had well-controlled symptoms within the prior month, there was no benefit (to invasive procedures)," study chair Dr. Judith Hochman told TCTMD.com. "So, I really can't see why people would still be recommending an invasive strategy, stenting, or bypass surgery, and I would think that the number of those procedures would decrease."

That decrease remains to be seen. Currently, there are about one million cardiac stent procedures done in the U.S. every year, costing about $30,000 a pop. And the 160,000 or so bypass operations can cost $100,000 or more. It all adds up to about fifty billion reasons ($$$) why the medical establishment may be so resistant to chelation therapy, which seems capable of opening up arteries or detouring blood flow in a safer manner at a fraction of the cost.

"If everyone who had heart disease went through a year's worth of chelation before undergoing open-heart surgery or a stent, we would effectively reduce the number of procedures by at least 25 percent, and probably a lot more," says former heart surgeon Dr. Robert Willix. "If we took away 25 percent of the revenue from cardiovascular disease in the United States, they'd have to close 50 percent of those hospitals, because it's the No. 1 money-making proposition for hospitals."

In addition to the procedures themselves, a patient typically has to undergo a battery of tests, which may include any or all of the following: blood tests, electrocardiogram (EKG), stress test, nuclear stress test, echocardiogram (ultrasound), coronary angiogram, magnetic resonance imaging (MRI), and coronary computed tomography angiogram (a type of CT scan). These all help to determine if there is any blockage in coronary arteries and, if so, where they are located and how severe the ischemia. As you might imagine, these tests add a lot of cost to the treatment of heart disease.

Surgeries and stents basically deal with the heart's plumbing. And while problem spots can be opened up or bypassed, the procedures don't do anything to fix the underlying problem of atherosclerosis. That's one reason why the standard of care for heart disease also includes some pharmaceutical drugs, such as those designed to treat hypertension and high cholesterol. The hypertension drugs lower blood pressure, protecting arteries from the damage it can cause. And the cholesterol drugs inhibit the production of fatty substances that accumulate in plaque. Some of the most widely prescribed drugs in the U.S. are cholesterol-lowering statins, such as Lipitor, Crestor, and Zocor. In 2003, Lipitor became the best-selling drug of all time. And the total sales of statins, since they first hit the market in the late 1980s, have now surpassed $1 trillion.

They mostly work by disabling an enzyme in the liver that produces cholesterol and are heralded for not only reducing "bad" LDL cholesterol and triglyceride levels, but also for increasing "good" HDL cholesterol production, stabilizing arterial plaque so it doesn't rupture and cause blood clots, and reducing inflammation.

"Statins are the 'gold-standard' for high cholesterol treatment," proclaim experts at UT Southwestern Medical Center on its website. "They're a powerful medication, and they've been proven to save the lives of many men and women living with, or having a high risk of, heart attack or stroke."

And TACT director Dr. Lamas says the ISCHEMIA study "should make all of us (cardiologists) mindful that the medicines we are using, including aspirin, statins, beta-blockers, ace inhibitors, and angiotensin receptor blockers, really do have a tremendous effect retarding the progression of atherosclerosis. One day I hope that chelation will be part of that, but it really will depend on the studies that are being done now."

Still, critics contend that the benefits of statins have been grossly overblown, especially for people with "high cholesterol" but no symptoms of heart disease.

"After twenty-five years of statin research, the best of the studies shows that in primary prevention (people with no history of heart disease), statins have approximately 1 percent, or less, improvement in strokes, heart attack, and mortality," notes Dr. Brownstein, author of fifteen books including *The Statin Disaster*. "In secondary prevention, where someone has already had a cardiac event and is trying to prevent another one, the studies show no reduction in mortality and about a 3 percent reduction in non-fatal strokes and heart attacks. That means that either 99 or 97 percent of the people who take statins get no benefit from them."

Not surprisingly, other studies claim the exact opposite. Perhaps the most dramatic was the 2008 Justification for the Use of Statins in Primary Prevention: Intervention Trial Evaluating Rosuvastatin (JUPITER), which was published in the esteemed *New England Journal of Medicine*.

The data suggest a 54 percent heart attack risk reduction and a 48 percent stroke risk reduction in people at risk for heart disease who used statins as preventive medicine. However, that study came under a blistering attack in a "critical reappraisal" published in *The Annals of Internal Medicine*. It was blasted primarily for bias, which is understandable seeing how the study was funded by AstraZeneca, producers of Crestor, the brand name of rosuvastatin, and one of the more widely prescribed statins.

Of course, just because a pharmaceutical company with a vested interest sponsored the study doesn't mean the results should be summarily discounted. The same goes for the fact that nine of the fourteen authors had financial ties to AstraZeneca, and the two principal investigators had other conflicts of interest.

Still, you have to wonder how all of those entanglements may have affected the outcome. Truth is, a majority of clinical drug trials are funded by pharmaceutical companies and often carried out at institutions with financial ties to the companies.

Of course, I'm cherry-picking the studies. It's easy to do and you really can find a study to support pretty much any point you want to make. I picked JUPITER because it's such a good example of what's wrong in the whole system.

The Bottom Line

The bottom line to all of this is that it's very hard to know what to believe. It's a mark of our times. The more information we have at our disposal, the more difficult it is to separate fact from conjecture. Reality, which seemed easy to define just a generation ago, has become nebulous.

To their credit, conventional doctors want to feel assured that the treatments they offer patients are both safe and effective, and their guideposts have long been these gold-standard trials performed under a stringent set of guidelines that are designed to make them as objective and accurate as possible.

In a perfect world, the results of the trials would be sacrosanct. Sadly, it is not a perfect world. While the studies can offer some degree of assurance about a drug or procedure, they should not be relied upon for definitive proof.

"Physicians want to see the data to support what we do," explains cardiologist Dr. Larry Dean, Director of the University of Washington Medicine Regional Heart Center. "Getting data on everything we do is not easy, or even possible, and we often have to make decisions based on less-than-adequate information. There is no perfect study. They all have warts. That's why one study doesn't prove a point. But at the end of the day, when you look at all of the evidence from a body of studies, you have to be willing to accept what the literature says."

On the other hand, you can't dismiss the experiences of ordinary people in real-world situations. The folks getting chelation treatments in the Born Clinic and other facilities like it around the country are a living, real-time laboratory. They report seemingly miraculous things with a surprising consistency, seeing benefits not only for themselves but for so many others. It's really hard to find anyone who's had chelation therapy say anything bad about it.

That's not to say the current standard of care for heart disease—surgical procedures and drug therapies—is no good for anyone. My own father had heart disease, suffering his first attack at age forty-three. That one was relatively mild and called "a warning" by doctors. A decade later, while boating on the Chesapeake, he had a massive heart attack that nearly killed him. But a folksy doctor in a small Elkton, Maryland, hospital saved his life with a shot of epinephrine right through his breastbone to jump-start his heart. In his sixties, my dad had another devastating attack on the evening before he was scheduled for a bypass operation. Luckily, he was in the hospital for the prep when his heart stopped. A crackerjack orderly performed CPR to keep the blood flowing, and an emergency bypass operation brought him back from the dead. He finally succumbed to stomach cancer at age seventy-two. His heart continued to beat strongly in his final days, so much so we wished it would just give out to end his suffering. Without CABG surgery and drugs, there's little question my father wouldn't have lived that long. And until the cancer hit, he was active, mentally sharp, and otherwise had a very good quality of life.

On the other hand, my father never sought any type of therapy outside of the conventional. And the current standard of care may not be the best answer for everyone, as shown in the next chapter, when we examine the chelation option.

IN THEIR OWN WORDS

I had aching and pain but didn't know what it was. I went to a heart doctor, and he gave me Lipitor, which just made me feel worse. My legs were hurting. I couldn't lift my arms. I had circles under my eyes. So I went to see Dr. Trowbridge, and he said I had rheumatoid arthritis. He gave me chelation and vitamins. My RF (Rheumatoid Factor) was 400 but dropped down to 98 and then bounced back to a little over 100, which is still really high. But at least I feel like a human being again. I chelate every three weeks.

It's given me a new life. It's given me energy and everything I need as an old lady. Our bodies deteriorate as we get older, but chelation has kept it at bay so that I can move without pain. I thank the Lord for that, and Dr. T, too. He saved my life.

Nancy L., 78, Conroe, Texas

CHAPTER 8

Is Chelation a Good Option for Your Heart Disease?

When Eugene Wisenbaker was forty-eight years old, he was awakened early one Monday morning by the crushing pain of a heart attack. He went to the hospital, where doctors performed an angioplasty to open up the stricken blood vessels, then implanted two stents to keep them that way.

"I have to admit the doctors got me out of a jam, but that's as far as it went," says Eugene, now seventy years old. "The cardiologists I saw after that didn't have a clue how to keep me out of the hospital. I had nine more episodes over the next two years, and I needed to go to the emergency room with blood pressure as high as 220 over 146."

While those nine episodes were likely caused by transient problems that passed rather than full-blown heart attacks, they were still life-threatening. Making matters worse, Eugene had no insurance and wound up leaving the hospital after a few hours against doctors' orders.

"Each time I walked out, I had to sign a release saying I was aware I could die," he recalls. "The last time, I was in Galveston, Texas, and I almost didn't make it out of there alive. They told me they reached for the paddles to bring me back but were able to put some kind of medicine into the IV to revive me. A couple of hours later, I signed another release and walked out of the hospital, again being told I could die.

"On the way home, I said to my wife, 'Baby, I have *got* to find something different.'"

His first stab at an alternative came after he met a Native American medicine man at a café.

"For nearly two years, I'd been going into the hospital every six weeks like clockwork," he says. "That medicine man gave me some herbs and things that broke the six-week cycle. I went more than two and a half months without an episode and thought to myself, 'Maybe there is something to this alternative medicine stuff.'"

Later, a compounding pharmacist in Houston gave him "a concoction," including B-complex vitamins and niacin, that he says helped to reduce his cholesterol.

"The pharmacist told me I had to go see Dr. Trowbridge, who does chelation therapy," says Eugene. "I had no idea what that was, but I was desperate. The pain in my chest was so bad at times I couldn't raise my arms over my head.

"Well, I started seeing Dr. T, and after the third chelation treatment, my chest pain went away and never came back. I did it once a week for over five years, and my heart kept getting stronger and stronger. I slowed down after that and wound up with some blockages in my legs. But when I went to a cardiologist who did scans and ultrasounds and whatnot, he said my heart's clean as a whistle."

Eugene believes chelation also helped him cognitively. After his heart troubles began, he says his mind used to "lock up" on occasion.

"I'd be paying bills and suddenly I didn't know what I was doing," says Eugene, who owns and operates a florist shop with his wife.

He also plays the tenor saxophone, and the brain fog was so bad he had trouble picking up rhythm patterns.

"After doing chelation for a couple of years, it was a lot easier to get into the music," he says. "These days, I play gigs with the church orchestra. I'm as active as I've ever been. Without chelation, I wouldn't be here today. I can say that for a fact."

How Chelation Works for Heart Disease

Eugene is fairly typical of the chelation heart patients I interviewed for this book. Like him, they tend to be wary of conventional medicine despite the fact that at one time in their medical adventures, a conventional procedure probably saved their lives, like the doctors who got Eugene "out of a jam" during his first trip to the hospital. A lot of the patients started chelation after having had stents and bypasses, which means their heart disease was pretty advanced. Even with chelation treatments, some still needed medication and maybe even another procedure or two. Others, like Eugene, seemed to walk away from heart disease and never looked back.

"I had two patients removed from the heart transplant list because they improved so much," says Trowbridge. "That sounds to me like a pretty good treatment compared to a heart transplant. Here's the funny thing: I can't put them on or take them off the list. The doctors downtown did that after watching the patients get better. And how many of them do you think called me to say, 'What are you doing?' None. Not one."

Dr. Tammy Born says the results somewhat depend on what condition the patients are in when they start chelation. "If it's early in the progression of their disease, they generally do better," she notes. "Others who have more advanced conditions have a harder time. A lot of the people we see come here as a last resort, after everything else has failed. Chelation is a great tool, but we can only do so much."

In the previous chapter, we discussed the standards of conventional care for heart disease, which primarily consist of stents, bypass surgery, and medications. Basically, they are ways to deal with atherosclerosis, the narrowing of arteries due to plaque as we age. Chelation is another option, or perhaps addition, to the standard care. By lowering the toxic load of heavy metals in the body, chelation therapy can help reverse atherosclerosis.

The reason why is complicated and not fully understood. But here's what we know in a nutshell. Heavy metals stimulate production of free radicals called reactive oxygen species (ROS), which are unstable molecules that overwhelm the natural antioxidant defense system in cells. ROS cause oxidative stress, and that triggers an accumulation of cellular waste, most notably advanced glycation end products (AGEs) that are a byproduct of burning glucose for energy. That, in turn, causes inflammation, which promotes just about any disease you can name.

Inflammation in blood vessels causes plaque buildup because it creates fertile ground for the accumulation of cholesterol, calcium, the clotting agent fibrin, and other substances that circulate in the bloodstream. The stiffening and narrowing of the arteries not only restrict blood flow but also raise blood pressure, which further inflames and damages the delicate lining of the vessels.

By removing calcium and heavy metals from blood vessel cells, the vessels become less rigid. Blood flow improves, blood pressure drops, and the likelihood of plaque deposits getting thicker or rupturing diminishes. In fact, plaque buildup often shrinks dramatically.

"I've seen calcium scores (in coronary arteries) go down with chelation," says integrative physician Dr. David Brownstein. "I've seen carotid arteries go from 90 percent blocked down to less than 10 percent."

The exact mechanism explaining why blood vessel health is improved through chelation is still being debated. The so-called "calcium hypothesis" is based on EDTA's ability to latch onto calcium molecules in the bloodstream and shepherd them to the kidneys for elimination from the body. That creates a blood-calcium deficit. Because the body is programmed to remain in homeostasis—stability—hormonal reactions trigger the release of calcium from tissue. Ultimately, that comes not from bone and teeth, where the calcium is needed, but from places where it isn't needed, such as arthritic joints, kidney stones, and the plaque in blood vessels.

Besides contributing to the narrowing of blood vessels, calcium also acts as a cementing agent that binds together all of the other gunk clogging up the arteries. So once its level is reduced, the other molecules can be more easily swept away by the flow of blood through the vessels.

Another theory, called the "heavy metal hypothesis" focuses on chelation's ability to remove toxic heavy metals from tissue. Cells that were impeded by the metals are revitalized, and they become more efficient at optimizing circulation.

"EDTA is an excellent antioxidant that reduces oxidative stress," explains former heart surgeon Dr. Robert Willix. "It reduces inflammation, particularly in the micro-capillaries, and that increases collateral circulation. The heart gets blood flow that it wasn't getting before. In effect, EDTA chelation does a lot of what bypass surgery does without cutting people open."

Other theories include EDTA's blood-thinning capabilities. Making platelets "less sticky" not only helps to keep your blood test samples from clotting (remember, a form of EDTA is used in blood test collection tubes), but also the blood remaining in your body. Blood clots typically cause heart attacks and the most common type of strokes, among other things. Yet another theory is that EDTA boosts the body's production of nitric oxide, which relaxes and dilates blood vessels to improve flow.

Chelation versus Standards of Care

No matter what the mechanism, chelation takes longer to work than a bypass, and cardiologists tend to believe that people who chelate in a bid to avoid open heart surgery are foolishly risking their lives. But as we discovered in the previous chapter, bypass surgery is somewhat life-threatening in itself.

Willix speaks from experience as a cardiac surgeon. He was actually the first and only one performing open heart surgery in the state of South Dakota for a couple of years in the mid-1970s. But he soon decided that he was more interested in keeping people healthy than trying to fix them up after their bodies broke down.

"I'd always been athletic but had turned into a slug at age thirty-four," Willix recalls. "I decided to go vegan. Then I fell in love with running and did my first marathon in 1979. All of this led to me learning more and then teaching people how to prevent heart disease. A couple of years later, I quit surgery to focus on preventative medicine."

Chelation became one of Willix's go-to therapies despite the pushback from his former conventional colleagues. The main arguments against using chelation to prevent or treat heart disease is that there has been no definitive scientific proof it is both safe and effective. But given the sheer number of people who have been treated with EDTA chelation without adverse effects, it's a hard argument to make that it is not safe. The TACT 1 study alone involved more than 55,000 infusions, and there were more

PHYSICIAN PROFILE
DR. ROBERT WILLIX, JR.

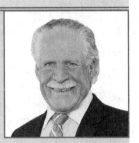

Enlightened Living Medicine, Palm Beach Gardens, Florida

Undergraduate: Boston College, Biology 1963

Medical School: University of Missouri, 1969

Specialty: Cardiac surgery, age management, energy medicine

Selected Honors and Associations:

- First Board-Certified Thoracic and Cardiovascular Surgeon in the State of South Dakota
- Kaul Foundation award for Pioneering in the field of Preventative Medicine
- Alan P. Mintz Award for Excellence in Age Management Medicine
- Chief Medical Officer for Hippocrates Health Institute
- Chief Medical Officer for Liquivida Lounge
- Member of the Board of Age Management Medicine Group
- Member of TEC – Chief Executives Working Together
- Mesa Holder – INKA Andean Shamanic Tradition
- Completed 14 marathons and more than 100 triathlons, including the 1984 Ironman in Kona, Hawaii
- Author of *The Rejuvenation Solution* (Simon & Schuster) and seven other books

Website: https://www.elmedicine.com/

Quote: "I believe that physicians have to become the model for their patients. I live the lifestyle I want my patients to live."

adverse reactions in the placebo group than the active drug group. Chelation's effectiveness may be more debatable, but certainly not to people like Eugene Wisenbaker, who believes it pulled him out of an endless cycle of ER visits.

Conversely, it's hard to prove that bypass surgery is either safe or effective. To date, there have been zero double-blind, placebo-controlled CABG studies. Obviously, it would be impossible to do a double-blind study because surgeons would know if they performed a bypass or not. And placebos are not viable. Who would agree to have their chest cracked open with just a fifty-fifty chance of actually having the bypass? As we discussed in the previous chapter, CABG is not very safe based on its mortality and complication rates, and its long-term effectiveness is also lacking, considering the relatively high percentage of patients who wind up needing another procedure eventually.

Despite the shortcomings of CABG surgery, Willix admits that it may sometimes be the best bet. In one case, a patient came to see him in the Boca Raton, Florida, health clinic he owned in the late 1980s.

"The man had a high-grade stenosis (narrowing) in the left anterior descending artery (LAD), which is also called the 'widow-maker,'" says Willix. "He had an 85 percent occlusion (blockage), but only one vessel was affected, and he was a relatively young guy in his fifties.

"I told him, 'Go have bypass surgery. It's too risky not to do it, and it will save your life.' But he was afraid of bypass and insisted I chelate him. I refused because I believed that bypass surgery was his best option. I said, 'Your wife is sitting here, and if I chelate you and something occurs, you're going to be dead and she's going to blame me. I won't do it.'

"Five years later, I'm at (the health food store) Wild Oats and this guy taps me on the shoulder. He says, 'You're a fraud.' I didn't recognize him, so he told me, 'I'm the guy you refused to chelate, but I went out and found someone who had the guts to do it. I chelated then, and I'm still doing it. My LAD lesion is smaller than it was then, and I'm still around, no thanks to you.'

"That was a wakeup call for me, and since then I never ever stop listening to my patients, because their intuition and innate knowledge of their own bodies is more important than anything a doctor knows."

Is Chelation Right for You?

I'm not sure most doctors would agree with Willix that patients know more than they do, or most patients for that matter. People tend to blindly trust their doctors, often not even bothering to ask exactly what is wrong with their body and if there's any way to fix it without drugs or surgeries.

Taking pills is easier than dieting or exercising or even chelating, which can be time-consuming. But if you've read this far in this book, you are likely someone who believes your health is more important than a temporary inconvenience. The question then becomes, is chelation right for you?

The short answer is that if you are diabetic or have heart disease (or even a family history of it), chelation is a no-brainer. Diabetics are prone to circulatory problems because the high sugar content in their blood promotes artery disease, at least in part by disabling an enzyme that protects the delicate endothelium cells lining the blood vessels. Heart patients, many of whom are also diabetic, have circulatory problems for a variety of reasons. And chelation reverses atherosclerosis with virtually no side effects, apart from a lightening of the wallet.

Because insurance companies have not yet figured out that chelation could literally save them billions of dollars spent on stents and bypass surgeries, it is not covered. So, the cost typically falls on you, the patient. The recommended twenty-session starter protocol will set you back anywhere from $2,000 to $5,000, which is a big chunk of change for most people. On the other hand, if your car needed a new transmission, you probably wouldn't think twice about coughing up that kind of dough to fix it, or spend even more for a new car, because you need it to get to work, the market, and your grandkids' soccer games.

Well, news flash, you need your body even more. And unlike a worn-out car, you can't just trade it in for a new one (at least not yet). Once you make the outlay for your initial chelation sessions, the once-a-month maintenance costs about as much as dinner for two at a nice restaurant. Eat out once a month less and you can afford the maintenance, which may keep you from having your chest ripped open or body parts amputated, or even delay being harvested by the Grim Reaper.

"You're Not Dead?"

One of Willix's favorite chelation stories is about a short, thin woman in her seventies who'd undergone bypass surgery five years earlier but had developed intractable angina.

"Women are tough to deal with because their blood vessels are much smaller than men's, especially in the heart," Willix says during an interview at the posh Hippocrates Health Institute in West Palm Beach, Florida, where he serves as Chief Medical Officer. "Her cardiologist had done all the things he could do to help her. But she continued to have chest pain and was popping nitroglycerin like candy, fifteen or twenty a day. The cardiologist finally threw his hands up in the air and said, 'Your vessels are so bad, and your ejection fraction is so low, I can't do anything else for you.'

"The woman was so bad off she couldn't walk a block. One of her sons knew me and brought her to my clinic, where I started chelating her. Within five treatments, she went from having trouble performing daily activities to doing chores around the house. After ten treatments, she no longer needed the nitroglycerin. A year later, this woman was walking four miles a day. She bumped into her cardiologist at a party, and he looked shocked to see her. He literally said, 'You're not dead?' She told him, 'Not only am I not dead, doctor, but I live an absolutely normal life.'

"She continued having monthly chelation treatments for five years before the angina came back. We upped her chelation but it didn't help at that point, and she died. But her sons thanked me because she had five good years that she wouldn't have had without chelation."

It should be noted that Willix is one of the integrative medicine practitioners who's been targeted by the Quackbusters, who continue to try to discredit alterative medical techniques and practitioners. But Willix seems proud to point out he's been on their "Quackwatch List." It's a badge of honor for him rather than a mark of shame because he is sure that he is on the right side of history.

Willix points out that the effects of chelation transcend having better circulation.

"One of the things chelation does, categorically, is it reduces angina attacks," he explains. "Usually by the tenth treatment, patients will tell you that they're no longer feeling chest pain as often as they were. And once you reduce that symptomology, they can go for the walk, or take the stairs, because these things no longer cause pain. They feel better, they do more, and they are more willing to listen to you when you tell them to change their lifestyle."

Getting the Lead Out

TACT study director Dr. Lamas chuckles when talking about lifestyle changes.

"None of my patients listen to my advice about diet," he says. "I just ask them not to be obese, or if they are obese, to get down to just being overweight. Fat is toxic."

However, heavy metals are even more toxic, with lead arguably being the biggest threat due to its stubborn pervasiveness in the environment, despite years of effort to rein it in. Lead not only damages blood vessels but also raises LDL cholesterol levels and promotes blood clots.

A 2017 study published in the *International Journal of Epidemiology* notes that deaths from cardiovascular disease dropped by 43 percent between the mid-1980s and the early 2000s. The drop could not be fully accounted for by improvements in reducing traditional risk factors, such as cholesterol and blood pressure levels. Experts concluded that nearly one-third of the decrease was likely due to reductions in environmental exposure to lead and its fellow heavy metal cadmium.

Still, Lamas says that we have a hundred times the amount of lead in our bones than the bones of ancient people. Lead initially enters red blood cells where it hangs out for a few months or less before settling into bone for its thirty-year half-life. That means it would take thirty years for your body to clear out half of its lead, if you weren't constantly absorbing more of it, which is impossible in the modern industrialized world.

Over the years, lead leaches out of bone as it remodels itself. The rate accelerates with the natural loss of bone density that comes with age. That puts lead back into the bloodstream, where it can wreak havoc on tissue throughout the body. According to Lamas, most older people have a lead blood level of at least one or two micrograms per deciliter, which is considered acceptable by the Environmental Protection Agency (EPA). But lead is extremely toxic to vascular tissue, particularly the delicate endothelium that lines the interior of the vessels.

Lead displaces essential minerals that are vital for intracellular reactions, causing dysfunction. Furthermore, it creates a lot of oxidative stress. Recent research suggests that lead also disrupts the histone proteins that spool and unspool DNA, meaning it messes with the way DNA controls genes. In general, "safe" levels of lead have been dropping over the years, with five micrograms per deciliter now being the threshold for adults. But a growing body of research suggests that there is really no safe level, especially for children.

"Lead and cadmium are poisons that have profound effects on human metabolism, potentially epigenetics and genetics," says Lamas. "They affect every aspect of the cell and every aspect of the cardiovascular tree."

Those effects were reflected in the TACT 1 study.

"Although I can't say we pinpointed the mechanism that led to the results, when you look at the event curve (subsequent heart problems), especially in the diabetic sub-group, it continued to separate after the therapy stopped," notes Lamas. "That strongly suggests that you have done something long-lasting. If you do that with statins, the curve starts going back together quickly (once the treatment is stopped). With chelation, it was as if a lifetime's accumulation of toxins was removed, and that turned you into a different biological unit. So now the likelihood of having something bad happen to you is less."

But he also cites evidence that suggests the mechanism for improving circulation rests with the removal of calcium from blood vessels.

"The question is: If the heavy metal hypothesis is true, then why do the patients with peripheral artery disease so quickly have an improvement?" Lamas muses. "Usually between the fifth and tenth infusion, you already know it is working. To me, that supports the calcium hypothesis, which is you're decalcifying the arterioles, making them a little more flexible so blood can flow more freely.

"I'm not sure whether the heavy metal hypothesis or calcium hypothesis will win out in the end. It might turn out to be a mix of mechanisms."

In a bid to find out, Lamas and his team are collecting heavy metals pre- and post-chelation in all TACT 2 patients. They are being stored in a biorepository, and the CDC is going to conduct a complex statistical analysis to try to determine if it is the removal of metals that caused the improvement of patients.

"It seems reasonable that you would have these effects by removing lead and other poisons from the body," says Lamas. "But you need the statistics to back it up.

"I am not a chelation clinician. I am a scientist trying to develop a new treatment for what I think is an unrecognized cardiovascular risk factor, similar to cholesterol before it was recognized as a risk factor in the Framingham study."

Nine Catheterizations and Four Stents

One person who doesn't need any statistics is Mark Bedsloe, a seventy-year-old businessman from Rochester, Michigan, who believes heavy metals contributed to his chronic heart disease.

"When I was tested, I had two or three times the acceptable level of lead and two other metals in my body," he says while undergoing a chelation infusion at the Born Clinic. "I got to thinking about the metals, and when I was a kid going to elementary school in downtown Detroit, industry was at its peak, and the chimneys were constantly pumping out black smoke. I remember before going outside for recess, we'd go into the bathroom and wet paper towels so we could wipe the soot off of the jungle gym, swings, and everything before playing on them. I'm speculating now, but that may be how the metals initially got into my system."

Mark says he's had a heart murmur since birth, and at age eleven he was stricken with rheumatic fever, which can damage the heart. Still, he was always athletic and active. But in 1999, at age fifty, he had a heart attack that required two stents.

"They told me they'd cleaned me out and I'd be good to go for twenty years," he says. "But I had another blockage in three years, then another in two years, then after one year, then after six months. Long story short, in ten years I had nine catheterizations and four stents."

Things changed for Mark in 2009 when he went to watch a hydroplane race with his son Patrick, who brought along his best friend, Drew Born, the doctor's son.

"Drew said you ought to see my mom," recalls Mark. "I did, and she put me on a very intense chelation program, doing three infusions a week for a year. To say I felt better is an understatement. Even my skin, which was grayish, got its color back to the point that my friends all kept asking me if I'd been to Florida.

"And it really helped me emotionally. For ten years I'd go to bed every night wondering if I was going to wake up. Whenever I said goodbye to my wife and kids, I'd wonder if I was ever going to see them again. Dr. Born took all of those fears away, and I can't put into words how that makes me feel."

Doing better, he slacked off on driving two and a half hours from his home to the Born Clinic once a month for maintenance treatments, and in February 2019 he needed open heart surgery.

"Dr. Born was always realistic about my condition," he says. "She told me the chelation was helping but that I had coronary heart disease and it's eventually going to come back. The doctors would have just put another stent in, but they couldn't because the blockage was at a 'Y' where two vessels came together. Now I'm back on schedule with the chelation and feel great. I've always been an avid cyclist and had to lay off for six months after my surgery. But I just did a seventy-mile ride. People ask me why I did it, and I tell them, 'Because I can.'

"I believe Dr. Born is an angel from heaven sent to me at just the right time. I don't have the words to express my appreciation for her."

These days, he has added motivation to make that long drive for chelation every month. His son Patrick is now the Born Clinic's business manager.

"It's a great excuse to see Patrick," says Mark. "I love living my life. My health scares have actually made me appreciate it more."

Chelation for Prevention

You might paraphrase Ben Franklin in saying, "A gram and a half of EDTA is worth a pound of stents and bypass grafts."

That's the amount of the drug that is typically infused during a chelation session, and there are plenty of people who would rather make that investment in time and money to prevent developing heart disease down the line.

Helen Higdon's father had several heart attacks and her mom died of heart failure, so she started getting chelation treatments from Dr. John Parks Trowbridge in the 1990s after reading a book about how it can prevent heart disease.

"I'm eighty now, my health is excellent, and I don't have symptoms of anything," says Helen, a retired elementary school teacher who still teaches Bible classes at her church in Kingwood, Texas. "Chelation gives me energy. I used to tell my husband, 'I chelated today, so you better stay out of my way or I'll run you down.'"

She even convinced her brother to do it. But after about seven years, he got too busy and quit.

"Nine months later, he called me and said he was going in for a quadruple bypass," Helen recalls. "I told him I knew this would happen and urged him to go back to chelation. But he did the bypass instead and died four years later. As far as I'm concerned, he killed himself by not sticking with chelation. If you have heart problems in your family, it would behoove you to do chelation, and don't stop it.

"I do it every month, without fail, and I don't have a pain in my body. I don't know what pain is, but I pray for people who have it."

Dr. Born believes that preventative chelation treatments are needed now more than ever.

"Every person I test has heavy metals in their bodies, and when you combine that with the overload of herbicides, pesticides, hormones, antibiotics, and other things we are getting exposed to, it lowers the threshold for disease," she says. "Chelation can at least remove the heavy metals, which lightens the load on our biological defenses. In a perfect world, everyone over forty would be chelated. It should be a regular thing, like getting your teeth cleaned."

IN THEIR OWN WORDS

I heard about chelation through a friend who's a chemist and was doing the oral version. I'd had a double bypass in my forties, but I was in my seventies then [when my friend did the oral version] and there was nothing wrong with me. I read up on chelation, and it all sounded very good. I did the IV version a couple of times a month, maybe fifteen or twenty times in all. I didn't like sitting there for two or three hours with nothing to do but read or watch TV. I don't know if it did anything or not. Doctors all say it's a scam. I can't argue it one way or another. It didn't have any bad effects. Maybe it's helped me to keep going for eighty-eight years, maybe not.

Bob L., Hatboro, Pennsylvania

CHAPTER 9

Chelation and Blocked Blood Flow

In his youth, Carlos Perez was a well-known baseball pitcher in Cuba.

"I was always athletic and represented Cuba internationally," he says. "I was offered a contract to play baseball professionally, but I didn't want that."

Instead, he went into his family's pineapple-exporting business, but came to the States in the early 1960s to escape Fidel Castro's dictatorship. With $27 and a dream, he started importing bananas from Costa Rico and Colombia and built his company, Banana Services, Inc., into a multimillion-dollar business.

Carlos served on the National Advisory Council of the Small Business Administration, and in 1984 was one of five Americans declared to be "Heroes for the '80s" by President Ronald Reagan. Since then, he's served as a Miami radio personality, rallying his fellow Cuban-Americans to support the drive for democracy in his stubbornly communist homeland.

But his health took a hit in 2015, when he was diagnosed with prostate cancer.

"They treated me with radiation, and I think it created a lot of free radicals that damaged my health," he says. "About six months later, I was exercising in the yard and told my wife I was feeling weak. She took me to the hospital, and they discovered I was having a heart attack."

Doctors implanted two stents in blocked coronary arteries. He was also diagnosed with peripheral artery disease, and another stent was implanted in his left leg to facilitate blood flow to the limb. The doctors said he'd need a stent in his right leg as well.

"After that, I could hardly walk," recalls Carlos. "My legs didn't seem to work right, and I was always short of breath."

Coincidentally, he read an article about chelation therapy in the *Miami Herald* and thought it may be able to help him. Dr. Lamas was quoted in the story, so Carlos called him up and began undergoing chelation treatments.

"I went once a week, and after the fifth or sixth session, I started walking better," he says. "From that point on, I improved dramatically."

In all, Carlos figures he's had between sixty and seventy chelation infusions. He also adjusted his diet, eating less meat and more monounsaturated fats.

He never got that stent for his right leg, and at eighty-seven years old, he doesn't seem to miss it.

"I walk between four and five miles every day, in all weather," says Carlos, who strolls the streets near his home in Coral Gables, Florida. "I've been doing it for a few years now, and I have no plans to stop."

Amazing "Feet"

During the TACT 1 study, Dr. Lamas got to know practitioners he may have once accused of quackery. His opinion changed, especially after the study was unblinded in 2012.

"The positive results were unexpected to me, but they weren't unexpected to my colleagues in the chelation community," he confesses. "They expected all along that the trial would be positive, but still breathed a sigh of relief. Meanwhile, they told me, 'You have to do a study on peripheral artery disease.'"

So, Lamas procured funding for a pilot peripheral artery disease study from Mount Sinai Medical Center and the James Carter Memorial Fund. The study selected only severe cases, where the patients had critical limb ischemia, a condition in which blocked blood flow causes extreme pain and/or diseased tissue. Diabetics with critical limb ischemia have a 25 percent annual risk of cardiovascular death and a 30 percent risk of amputation. Each patient in the trial was slated to get fifty infusions of the same disodium EDTA solution used in the TACT 1 studies over the course of a year.

"We had ten patients," says Lamas. "Three of them ended up getting amputations because they had such severe pain, they couldn't stick with the program for even one month, which is generally how long it takes for the treatments to start working. The remaining seven all received more than twenty infusions, and no one had anything amputated. No one had a heart attack or anything else. They're all okay."

One of those patients was David Wallack, a longtime diabetic with a critical limb ischemia who agreed to be unmasked so his story could be told in this book. The condition caused him agonizing neuropathy pain and had turned parts of his left foot gangrenous. The results of his treatments are no less than extraordinary, as shown in a series of photos that Lamas used in a report of the study, which can be found at the following website: www.HumanixBooks.com/Chelation.

Perhaps there is no better testament to the power of chelation than actually seeing blackened tissue turn pink again right in front of your eyes.

"People can't see what happens to arteries in the heart, but people can see what happens to a diabetic foot," notes David's wife, Holly Wallack, who speaks for her eighty-three-year-old husband because he also has some short-term memory issues. "His foot was dying. The lesions were black and necrotic. After a year and a half of weekly chelation, you can look at both of his feet, and you can't tell which one had the problem."

David has been an insulin-dependent diabetic since the age of thirty-eight, but Holly says he managed it well until about three years ago when his left foot "became cold" and "changed color."

It turned out that he had an occlusion of the external iliac artery, the main blood supplier to the leg. Holly says a "brilliant" surgeon fixed that impasse, and David was okay for about a year. Then his femoral artery, which is a continuation of the external iliac, got clogged. A second operation by the same surgeon cleared that obstruction, but three of the four main arteries below the knee also had blockages.

"In layman's terms, all of the soot that was sitting in the blood vessels got pushed down to the foot after the second surgery, and there wasn't enough pressure to bring it back up and out," explains Holly. "He ended up with seven lesions on his foot, and the neuropathic pain was terrible. At that point, the surgeon said that the only option left was amputation."

That's not an unusual prognosis for diabetics. According to the American Diabetes Association, someone in the world loses a limb due to diabetes-related complications every thirty seconds, including about 200,000 Americans a year. Surveys suggest that as many as one in ten diabetics will develop lesions, and of those, as many as one in four will require amputations. Frighteningly, patients often need multiple surgeries as the doctors try to remove as little tissue as possible at first, only to return to cut off more when wounds don't heal or additional flesh turns gangrenous due to compromised circulation.

"After the surgeon said my husband would need to have his leg amputated below the knee, we went to a wound specialist at the University of Miami," recalls Holly. "She walked into the examination room, took one look at my husband's foot, and ran her finger across her throat, implying that it would have to be cut off. I said, 'Can't we at least try something else?'"

They tried hyperbaric oxygen therapy, which is designed to dramatically increase oxygen levels in the blood to repair tissue and restore function. But that didn't help. A second option was chelation therapy. Holly had heard about it from a friend whose husband had undergone chelation after suffering a massive heart attack at a very young age. The Wallacks were lucky enough to live in Miami Beach, not far from where Lamas and his TACT studies are based.

"With amputation as the only other option, I figured: What do we have to lose?" says Holly, a retired medical records advocate. "I knew that Dr. Lamas had done a study on chelation for heart patients at Mount Sinai, and they were looking for ten diabetic patients with peripheral artery disease for another study. So, it was a case of being in the right place at the right time."

Along with weekly EDTA infusions, David's wounds were meticulously cared for.

"We had to keep his foot completely dry and change the bandages every day," says Holly. "It was a very slow process. The lesions are like a scab when you scrape your knee, and the scab gets smaller as the skin beneath it heals. The wound-care surgeon would debride the lesions every other week, removing the scab around the edges and stimulating the growth of the healthy skin nearby. We did that for eighteen months, until there was just healthy tissue left."

There's little doubt in Holly's mind that chelation was the reason David's foot came back from the dead.

"He takes the same drugs he's been taking for many years," she says. "We changed nothing other than reducing the pain medication he took for the neuropathy from 150 milligrams twice a day to 25 milligrams once a day, which he probably doesn't even need since he has no pain.

"I've been in the medical field for quite some time, and I can tell you there can be no reason his foot healed other than chelation therapy."

Even though his foot is better, David continues to have weekly chelation infusions because it also seems to be improving his cognition. Holly says it's helped his memory a bit but really shows in his gait and ability to get around.

"Chelation isn't targeted therapy," she explains. "So if it's clearing the arteries in the heart as the TACT study shows, the arteries in the brain are getting clearer, and the arteries in the legs are getting clearer. The arteries everywhere are getting clearer."

Holly has been so impressed with the healing power of chelation that she was slated to start undergoing treatments herself just a few days after she told me her husband's story.

"I'm healthy, but I'm getting older, and the aging process causes me some memory problems," she admits. "I asked Dr. Lamas if I would benefit from chelation, and I'll never forget his answer. He said, 'I love my wife. I gave her twenty-five treatments.'"

CHELATION AND DIABETES

When heavy metals aren't corralled and spirited out of the body, they displace some of the essential minerals needed to complete enzymatic reactions. For example, zinc is needed for the synthesis and secretion of insulin from pancreatic cells. But zinc can get displaced by heavy metals, especially cadmium and lead. Zinc is not only vital in the production of insulin but also its reabsorption into the body. That task is carried out by an insulin-degrading enzyme, which breaks down the hormone after it ushers glucose from the bloodstream into the cell. If the hormone is not broken down, it stays in the bloodstream and the insulin receptors in the cells become less sensitive to it. That, in turn, can result in insulin resistance, which leads to diabetes. Once you get rid of the heavy metals, the enzymes can start processing insulin properly, taking at least one destructive factor out of the diabetes equation.

TACT 3a

Lamas and colleagues wrote a case report based on David's incredible turnaround, identifying him only as a male participant in the study. Surprisingly, he says he had trouble finding a medical journal in which to publish the results.

"The reviews came back saying, 'Well, did you image the arteries, or measure the flow?'" he recalls. "I felt like telling them, 'That patient was scheduled for amputation, and the foot's still on. It is pink and doesn't hurt. What more do you need?'"

Eventually, the case study was published in *Vascular Disease Management*. Lamas also presented the study at two events, the International Symposium of Endovascular Therapy in January

2019 and the Amputation Prevention Symposium the following August.

"Those two organizations don't have an anti-chelation bias," notes Lamas. "But even after presenting this case report to a receptive audience, no one from either of these organizations is doing chelation to save limbs. The only ones doing it are a bunch of alternative medicine people and me. I mean, what's up with that?

"Carlos Perez talks about chelation on his radio show every week. Meanwhile, people are losing legs in Miami every day, and I don't even get a phone call.

"So far as I know, if you're looking at conventionally trained cardiologists who use chelation, or are even studying it, as a tool to prevent heart attacks or amputations, I'm the only one. It's shocking and upsetting."

One of the attendees of the Endovascular symposium was Dr. Frank Veith, a pioneering vascular surgeon affiliated with both the Cleveland Clinic and New York University's Langone Medical Center.

"I thought Dr. Lamas' data were convincing," he says. "Chelation has been the 'bad boy' of treatment for many years, but I think there may be something there. At least he is treating it scientifically.

"Still, I'm a little skeptical. Sometimes, these things heal on their own. In the 1980s, we published a paper on patients with limited gangrene who got better without any treatment. But I believe it's important to evaluate new things, and just because someone else says they are smoke and mirrors, doesn't mean that they are."

Veith is even more skeptical that chelation can help people like Carlos Perez and Dr. Born's patient, Roman Rabiej, who suffered from intermittent claudication.

"That's *mishegoss*," he says. "No treatment helps claudication. Angioplasty, stents, and bypass may help symptoms for a little while, but eventually the treatment fails. The disease progresses, or the artery scars down and occludes again."

I tell him how chelation practitioners claim that EDTA can remove plaque from arteries without the trauma of those invasive procedures, but Veith isn't buying it—at least not yet.

"The best treatment for most vascular problems is no treatment, and prophylactic treatment doesn't work," he declares. "In fact, it sometimes can cause more complications than benefits."

Still, Veith remains open-minded enough to have invited Lamas to speak at his 2019 VEITHsymposium, a five-day event featuring the latest advances in treating vascular disease.

"He declined, though it wasn't anything malignant," notes Veith. "We'll try again next year."

By then, Lamas may have more data to convince the skeptics.

"With evidence from that ten-patient study, we were able to acquire enough money to do a fifty-patient randomized trial," he says. "I call it TACT 3a because I'm expecting to do a TACT 3, which will be a chelation study with two to three hundred patients who have severe peripheral artery disease."

In 2019, he began enrolling diabetics with critical limb ischemia for the fifty-patient study, some of whom already have gangrene. Like the previous TACT studies, it will be randomized, double-blind, and placebo-controlled. One problem is that about half of the participants will be getting the placebo, meaning their disease will likely progress. People in the placebo group could even lose limbs that might have been saved if they'd gotten the drug.

"It's like asking for randomized parachutists," laments Lamas. "But if you don't do a randomized trial, it won't be accepted by anyone. Top individuals from the peripheral artery disease world will serve on a safety monitoring board, and they will see unblinded data annually. They can stop a study if it becomes unethical to expose the patients to a therapy or, in this case, a placebo."

Meanwhile, his frustrations continue. Lamas and his team wrote a paper on the pilot study, which details the results for all ten patients. Once again, they had trouble publishing it and had to settle for the online journal *Cureus*.

"The pilot study was devilishly hard to publish," says Lamas. "We went to six journals, and they all wanted vascular flow data, ultrasound, and this and that, as if you didn't have a foot that stayed on rather than being amputated.

"There's the reality, and then there is the mechanism. I was just trying to establish the reality that using EDTA chelation for people with critical limb ischemia is worth pursuing. What we're doing now (TACT 3a) will look at mechanisms.

"To refuse to put this study into a traditional cardiology journal because we didn't do innumerable tests to show that the blood vessel flow was better, when that foot was about to be cut off, is nuts. It's a misuse of scientific thinking.

"I am a scientist, and my mind remains open. I don't discount the evidence I see with my own eyes, but I also can't discount the scientific process needed to prove it one way or the other."

CHAPTER 10

Chelation and the Fight Against Cancer

Judie McCallum was diagnosed with ovarian cancer in 2010.
"The doctors told me that if I didn't have chemo, surgery, and a complete hysterectomy, I'd be dead in a year," she says. "I refused it completely, and I still have all of my body parts. At seventy-six, I have no idea what I'm going to do with them, but I still have them."

Instead of the standard care, Judie chose to follow a self-administered protocol developed by the late Bill Henderson, author of *Cancer Free: Your Guide to Gentle, Non-Toxic Healing*. It consists of a plant-based diet, daily intake of cottage cheese and flaxseed oil, supplements, and lifestyle changes. For a while, Judie's cancer biomarkers went down. Then they began fluctuating, and in 2013 she discovered that the cancer was spreading into her colon.

Judie decided to enter a six-week program at Utopia Wellness, an Oldsmar, Florida, clinic run by Dr. Carlos Garcia, who co-authored the fourth edition of *Cancer Free*. The program includes EDTA chelation and other treatments. About four weeks into it, scans showed that Judie's cancer was gone. She remains cancer-free today but continues to be a regular at Utopia Wellness, not only attending to her own health but also helping to inspire others in their battle against cancer.

"I'm not the only one," says Judie, who lives in nearby Palm Harbor. "I've seen people come in here in wheelchairs with all kinds of cancer—pancreatic, breast, prostate, even brain cancers—and they eventually walk out on their own. I truly believe that if scientists did the right kind of research, they'd find that more people survive cancer with good quality holistic healing than surgery and chemotherapy."

"The Big C"

When I was young, I remember how people were reluctant to even utter the word "cancer," as if they could be stricken with the disease just by mentioning its name. Back then, "The Big C" was pretty much a death sentence. Some forms of it still are, like the glioblastoma brain tumor that took the life of Senator John McCain, an otherwise very durable guy. Odds are slim to beat that one.

Pancreatic cancer is also bad news, as is liver, stomach, lung, gall bladder . . . well, the truth is we haven't really come too far in finding that ever-elusive cure for cancer. And like heart disease, the failure has come despite hundreds of billions of dollars being invested in research, as well as the fact that a huge windfall awaits whatever pharmaceutical company can patent the cure.

Dr. Garcia will tell you that no one can find a cure for cancer because cancer is not an isolated problem, such as a staph infection or a broken bone, but rather a symptom of a sick body.

"Patients with cancer think it is a singular problem, compounded by all of the ramifications of ill-designed treatment programs such as chemotherapy," says Garcia, who treats a lot of cancer patients with alternative therapies at Utopia Wellness.

PHYSICIAN PROFILE
DR. CARLOS GARCIA

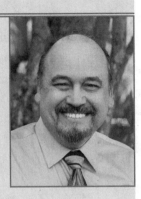

Utopia Wellness, Oldsmar, Florida

Undergraduate: University of Massachusetts, B.A., 1977

Medical School: University of Massachusetts, 1982

Specialty: Anesthesiology, Integrative medicine

Selected Memberships and Associations:

- American College of Pain Management – Diplomat
- American College for the Advancement of Medicine – Diplomat
- International College of Integrated Medicine
- University of Massachusetts Bilingual Collegiate Program
- International College of Integrative Medicine
- American Holistic Health Association

Website: https://utopiawellness.com

Quote: "A physician can only help you to the extent that you are willing to accept the help."

"The fact of the matter is that cancer is multi-faceted and may include circulatory, digestive, nutritional, dental, lifestyle, emotional, and other problems. You have to treat all of them, not just a tumor."

Garcia proudly wears a chip on his shoulder when it comes to conventional healthcare, which he calls "sick-care."

"The American healthcare myth is that once you get sick, you're always going to be sick," he says. "That's nonsense. If you change the paradigm of the body with the available therapeutic remedies, it will heal. You don't need pharmaceuticals, which do nothing to solve the underlying problems but manage to kill more than 10,000 Americans every month from adverse reactions."

He's not exaggerating. A 2016 investigation by *U.S. News & World Report* estimated that death by prescription drugs—taken as directed—is the fourth leading cause of mortality in this country. Oddly enough, we don't hear much about it.

Garcia was once an anesthesiologist whose life was upended when he slipped on an ice cube at home, fell down, and hurt his hand. He says an anesthesiologist with a bum right hand represents "a lawsuit waiting to happen," and the subsequent loss of his ability to acquire malpractice insurance led to him losing his job. He was sitting around wondering what to do with his life when a friend called and told him a local clinic needed a medical doctor to perform chelation therapy, which he knew nothing about at the time. But it didn't take long for him to appreciate its value.

"When I did chelation therapy on people, their blood pressure dropped, their need for diabetic medication dropped, their angina and peripheral neuropathy began to disappear, and we were able to save gangrenous organs," he recalls. "That inspired me to learn more about alternative therapies and redefine what medicine is supposed to be, which is the ability of the physician to help the body heal versus the illusion that drugs and procedures are going to cure you."

Garcia now claims that he can stop the progression of, and even reverse, many chronic diseases that are commonly considered incurable, including cardiovascular diseases, dementia, macular degeneration and others, using an array of therapies. But most of the people who come to his clinic suffer from late-stage cancer, and chelation therapy is a key element in bringing many of those patients back from the brink.

"Almost all of my patients are Stage IV and have been told to go home and die," says Garcia, who doesn't mince words. "After coming here, half of them live, half of them don't."

Virtually all of them get EDTA infusions to improve circulation, because oxygenated blood is one of a cancer cell's worst enemies. Cancer thrives in an anaerobic, acidic environment, which chelation reverses. Garcia explains it this way:

As vessels become clogged with arteriosclerotic plaque, blood flow diminishes. As blood flow diminishes, the amount of oxygen getting through to the cells diminishes. Cells use oxygen to generate energy. In order to survive the diminished blood flow, cells must start fermenting to generate energy. The fermentation process produces lactic acid, and the more acidic the cells become, the more dysfunctional they become. When you have EDTA chelation therapy, you start eliminating the calcium and other glues that hold the plaque together, and the body is able to remove it. Blood flow increases, cells get more oxygen, and they don't need to ferment to generate energy. Lactic acid decreases, the alkalinity of the cell increases, and function returns to normal.

Badda-bing, badda-boom. The cancer goes away.

Well, not really. Cancer is complicated, typically created by myriad factors that result in system-wide dysfunction. In general, conventional and alternative docs agree that you *do* have to throw the kitchen sink at this particular disease. But each sink holds different therapies. In the conventional world, surgery, chemo, and radiation are the mainstays. Even cutting-edge technologies, such as immunotherapies meant to induce the body's own defense system to attack cancer cells, may be effective in zapping the malignancy with less damage to healthy tissue, but they still don't address the cause. That's likely why so many cancers come back.

CHELATION PREVENTS CANCER IN SWISS

In 1958, a team of Swiss scientists embarked on a study of 231 adults who all lived in the same small city. Fifty-nine of them received ten or more injections of calcium EDTA, while the rest had no treatments. During an eighteen-year follow-up, only one of the fifty-nine (1.7 percent) who received the EDTA died from cancer. In contrast, 30 of the 172 (17.4 percent) who were untreated died of cancer. Both groups lived in the same neighborhood, adjacent to a heavily traveled highway. They were exposed to the same amount of lead from automobile exhaust, as well as industrial pollution and other carcinogens, levels that were similar to many other urban areas around the globe. Statistical analysis showed EDTA therapy to be the only significant difference between the two groups to explain the 90 percent reduction in cancer deaths.

The Alternative Toolbox

Garcia uses different tools, starting with diagnostics.

"People need to tell us what's wrong with them," he says. "Our job is to ask the questions. You give us answers, and with these answers we tell you what's going on and then choose from our armamentarium of therapies what to do for you."

Rather than relying primarily on blood tests, Garcia places a lot of emphasis on a Russian-made machine called Sensitiv Imago.

"It gives an analysis of what is going on electronically through people's organs so we can determine what is functioning and what is not functioning," he says. "The Russians are light years ahead of Americans with that kind of technology."

Once trouble spots are identified, a variety of treatments are chosen to attack these specific areas, including hyperbaric oxygen therapy; intravenous ozone, hydrogen peroxide, and nutrients; colon therapy; liver and gall bladder cleanses; FAR-infrared saunas; coffee enemas; herbs; tinctures; poultices, and more.

"Using single modalities will produce limited results," Garcia explains. "While all of the modalities I use are good in themselves, when you use them concurrently, the synergy between them makes each one more efficient than if it was just used alone. My clinic is like a mini-mall, so my patients don't have to shop around for different treatments at different places."

Pretty much every treatment plan calls for chelation, which jump-started Garcia into alternative medicine twenty-five years ago. He says he's now overseen some 80,000 infusions.

"I'm probably the world's most experienced chelator," he boasts.

In 2005, that attracted some attention from the FBI, as agents in full regalia raided his office and seized all of his records. Despite the scrutiny, he was allowed to continue practicing, and investigators ultimately could find no evidence of wrongdoing.

"Five years later, they returned all of my records and never presented me with a single charge," says Garcia. "I think the problem was that I had the largest chelation clinic in the country at the time. Basically, what I was doing was taking significant business away from the hospitals, which derive a lot of their income from stents, bypass operations, amputations, and the like."

Mind Games

Chelation is a uniquely social therapy. Just like at the Born Clinic, patients being chelated at Utopia Wellness typically sit together for a couple of hours at a time. They chat, get to know one another and offer support. And one day a week, they can engage in a counselor-led group therapy session.

"Toxic thoughts prevent healing," preaches clinic counselor Dan Mykins, a self-proclaimed "provocateur" and "agent of change" during a Wednesday morning session in December. "You need to learn how to give yourself unconditional love and trust."

'Tis the season for healing, as the IV EDTA bags hang alongside Christmas ornaments. It's a fitting juxtaposition, the pain, fear, and grief of the patients' potentially deadly conditions mingling with the hope, joy, and camaraderie that comes from connecting with others who not only understand their plight, but share it.

Tears are shed as patients talk about why they suppress their emotions or can't forgive themselves.

"You may hide your pain by laughing about it," Mykins tells one man who chuckled when describing his misfortunes. "But your body knows the truth. That's why you are here today. We're all pretty good at playing mind games, but you need to deal with your feelings honestly to heal. Relief comes from purging."

The purging ebbs and flows. Some patients are still not ready to recognize their problems, others remain unable to come to terms with them. But they see themselves in others, and that connection is enlightening, and comforting. Some, like Judie McCallum, have already emerged from the tunnel, and they offer inspiration to those who are still trying to find their way.

"I never really believed in talking to a psychologist because I knew I could do it all myself," says self-made businessman James Roberts III, a prostate cancer patient who goes by the name

Jimmy. "But in the group sessions, I could see in other people the same problem I had, and that helped me get over being so angry, confrontational, and impatient. I was finally able to open up about the problems I'd been carrying around."

Jimmy, who owns a national chain of outlets that recycle mobile home axles and tires, was diagnosed with his cancer in 2014 and went to the Cleveland Clinic for surgery in 2018. His PSA level (a biomarker for prostate cancer) initially fell after surgery but then began rising.

"I still don't know what was happening because the follow-up was practically non-existent," he says. "The surgeon moved to a different clinic, and I never got ahold of him, so I never found out exactly what he was able to get done. Meanwhile, I felt miserable. I had no energy and no will to do hardly anything."

His attorney's mother-in-law had found success with Garcia, so Jimmy flew to see him from his home in Van, Texas.

"Dr. Garcia told me the nagalase blood marker test that shows the amount of cancer I had in my body was nearly double some of his Stage IV patients," he says.

Through initially skeptical of alternative therapies, Jimmy stuck with Garcia's program through four three-week sessions. Along with chelation, he mentions having hyperbaric oxygen therapy, vitamin IVs, FAR infra-red saunas, lymphatic massages, and wave therapy, as well as dietary changes and group therapy.

"By the second week, I started feeling a little better, and by the end of the third I was feeling really good," he recalls. "Now, my PSA is lower, my liver function has improved, I was able to go off my high blood pressure medication, I'm sleeping better, and I've even got more hair growing back on my head.

"Dr. Garcia doesn't sugarcoat things. He tells you what's wrong and gives you options to fix it. But you have to take responsibility for your own health. It's not just going in there and letting them drip some medicine into your arm. Dr. Garcia will show you the way, but you have to fix yourself."

Garcia is a bit of a renegade, even among chelation practitioners. For example, he's not big on the popular monthly maintenance infusions, preferring his patients come back every two or three years for a dozen or so treatments.

"Plaque is like plaster, so one infusion doesn't do much to remove it," he explains. "You need several to loosen it up enough for the body to remove it."

But he agrees with the others on chelation's value to health. When asked if everybody should undergo chelation therapy, he replies: "If they're smart, they will."

CHAPTER 11

The Wide Range of Healing and Prevention Powers

Dr. Joe Hickey says he was a "straight-by-the-book" internist for the first twenty years he practiced medicine.

"It was statins for everybody as I tried to follow the rules," he notes. "But the diabetics started getting to me. Treating them was like sticking a finger in a dyke. No matter what I did, they ended up with problems springing up all over, and I felt like I wasn't really doing anything to help them."

When one of his patients went on the high-fat Atkins Diet, Hickey advised against it, saying he should instead be on a low-fat diet, which was more generally accepted at the time.

"The guy lost thirty pounds, and when I saw his bloodwork, I told him, 'Everything's great now that you're finally listening to me,'" Hickey recalls. "And he said, 'I'm actually not listening to you because I'm still on the Atkins Diet. You need to open your eyes and study it.'"

So he did, concentrating on its effect on lipids. His research revealed that eating healthy fats and cutting way down on carbohydrates optimized the size and density of the "bad" LDL cholesterol particles, a critical factor when it came to heart disease. He began putting patients on a high-fat, low-carb ketogenic diet.

"Their LDL particle size grew and became filled with fat instead of sugar (which made them less dense), and their heart disease improved," he says. "That was my first foray out of the box."

Then, in 2003, his cousin John was diagnosed with myelodysplastic syndrome, a deadly bone marrow disease.

"It's universally fatal," says Hickey. "Basically, his bone marrow stopped making blood cells. His hemoglobin, platelet, and white blood cell counts dropped dramatically. He became extremely anemic and turned ghostly white. At (the) Mount Sinai (bone marrow transplant center) in New York City, they checked him out and told him to 'get his affairs in order.' And when he went for a second opinion, the doctor stuck a needle in his hip, pulled out some bone marrow, and came back an hour later and said, 'Well, I won't be seeing you again.'"

A third consultation at Harvard got the same, though more diplomatic, response. So, John traveled from New York to Hilton Head, South Carolina, to see his doctor cousin Joe.

"I didn't think I could help him, but I prayed on it, and as we caught up he told me he'd been working as a plumber for the Indian Point nuclear power plant," says Hickey. "That struck me because I knew that plumbers sometimes have elevated lead exposure from their work (with lead pipes). And I knew that lead could cause anemia because it knocks iron and zinc out of the hemoglobin cascade, so you can't reproduce your blood."

Hickey didn't know much about metal toxicity or chelation, but he read up on them and began giving John three EDTA infusions a week.

"My internist partners started getting nervous when they saw an IV pole at the office and I told them I was chelating my

PHYSICIAN PROFILE
DR. JOE HICKEY

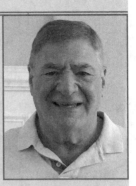

The Hickey Wellness Center, Hilton Head, South Carolina

Undergraduate: University of Notre Dame, 1973

Medical School: New York Medical College, 1977

Specialty: Integrative internist

Selected Honors and Associations:

- National Board of Medical Examiners, Diplomate
- International College of Integrative Medicine, Board Member
- Longtime featured physician on *Achieving Ultimate Health*, WLOW radio show
- Presenter/panel participant at numerous medical conferences
- Author of *Cholesterol Phobia! The Reason America Is Fat and Unhealthy*

Website: www.drjosephhickey.com/

Quote: "Once you remove heavy metals, the body knows how to heal itself. But you can't detox; you can't heal; you can't rejuvenate new tissue if there's this toxic block."

cousin," he says. "But I kept doing it, and after thirteen treatments his hemoglobin count almost doubled. After thirty treatments, his hemoglobin normalized. The myelodysplastic syndrome was completely reversed. John was supposed to be dead in 2004, and he's still alive, playing golf in Florida."

Wide-Ranging Healing Powers

John's story is a testament to the versatility of chelation. Still, it's likely not all people with myelodysplastic syndrome would be saved by it. The relationship between diseases and the human body is very complex, with a seemingly limitless number of variables. That's one reason why there probably will never be a universal cure for anything. Chelation helps by reducing one of those variables, heavy-metal toxicity, which in some cases may have dramatic effects. If certain genetics, chemicals, allergies, pathogens, or other factors are the primary cause of the disease, chelation may have less of an impact. That said, using chelation to reduce your toxic metal load is reputed to be potentially beneficial for a variety of conditions, including:

- Alzheimer's disease
- Amyotrophic lateral sclerosis (Lou Gehrig's disease)
- Angina pectoris
- Arthritis
- Atherosclerosis
- Autism
- Cancer
- Cataracts
- Chronic obstructive pulmonary disease (COPD)
- Coronary artery disease
- Depression
- Diabetes
- Erectile dysfunction
- Fibromyalgia
- Gangrene
- High cholesterol
- Hypertension
- Kidney stones

- Macular degeneration
- Multiple sclerosis
- Parkinson's disease
- Peripheral artery disease
- Post-traumatic shock disorder (PTSD)
- Psoriasis
- Thyroid disorders

We've already touched upon some cardiovascular-related conditions and cancer. The following is a look at a few others.

Depression and PTSD

After chelation infusions helped Dr. Hickey's cousin recover from a "universally fatal" disease, he started trying the therapy to treat other conditions.

"The next person was a mother of five who had a history of severe post-partum depression," he says. "She was so morbidly depressed she'd curl up into a fetal position. I sent her to every psychiatrist in the area, and they gave her different drugs. But nothing helped."

Hickey went back to the books. He found that heavy metals such as lead, mercury, cadmium, arsenic, and aluminum interfere with the brain's production of neurotransmitter proteins, including feel-good serotonin and anti-anxiety gamma-aminobutyric acid (GABA). To make them, magnesium is needed to catalyze certain enzymatic reactions. But heavy metals displace the magnesium, which disables the enzyme and halts production of the neurotransmitter proteins. With lower production of serotonin and GABA, a person is likely to feel sad and agitated, two common symptoms of depression.

Women have it particularly tough because they give calcium to fetuses when they are pregnant and lose bone mass at a higher rate than men after hitting menopause. In both cases, lead and other metals are freed from the bone tissue to wreak havoc on other parts of the body, including neurotransmitters, potentially causing depression and other mental problems.

"After reading a chapter about metals and neurotransmitters in a textbook, I asked my patient if she wanted to try chelation," says Hickey. "She told me she was ready to try anything at this point, so I chelated her and she got better. She's still fine more than ten years later, running around the island, happy as a lark."

Another patient, Robin Fulton, says she "had major PTSD (post-traumatic stress disorder) from sex abuse" that was exacerbated by a knee replacement and four other leg and toe surgeries over the course of three years.

"My world was closing in on me," says the sixty-two-year-old former tennis pro. "I was failing. I couldn't work. I couldn't think straight. I'd slur my words. I'd pick up a glass of water and my hand shook so much I thought I had Parkinson's. I had no interest in watching TV or listening to music. In short, I was like a vegetable."

She went to several doctors and no one could figure out how to help her. Finally, a friend suggested she see Hickey.

"He tested me and found out I had high levels of mercury, lead, and aluminum," she recalls. "So, I started chelation, and that was the catalyst for my rebirth."

That was ten years ago, and Robin says she was in such a fog back then she can't remember how long it took her to start feeling better. She figures she's undergone some eighty chelation treatments in the past decade and continues to get a few maintenance infusions every year. She's very active, though she traded tennis for hot yoga and other less impactful pursuits to save her legs the pounding. She's also found strength and stability through a type of mysticism that combines physics and consciousness, focusing on positive thoughts to reshape her once-shattered world.

"It's night and day," says Robin of her mental state. "I had one foot in the grave, and now I feel a thousand percent better. I call Dr. Hickey 'Saint Joe' because he saved my life."

Fibromyalgia

Next up for Hickey were fibromyalgia sufferers. Initially identified as a type of rheumatism, fibromyalgia syndrome, commonly referred to as fibro, wasn't recognized by the AMA as its own separate disease entity until 1987. It causes widespread pain in muscles and joints, along with tender spots that can trigger intense pain when pressed. Often, it is accompanied by chronic fatigue, sleeplessness, mood disorders, belly aches, headaches, and other symptoms.

Fibromyalgia, which affects mostly women, is also a disease of neurotransmitter function. Although people with fibromyalgia feel pain all over their bodies, it actually emanates from the spinal cord. The back of the spinal cord, called the dorsal horn, constantly produces serotonin and GABA to limit the pain response.

When you're exposed to a noxious stimulus—such as being stuck by a pin—an electrical impulse stops the production of serotonin and GABA, and a neuropeptide called substance P is released to tell the brain there was an injury in a certain area. People with fibro aren't making enough serotonin and GABA in the spinal cord, so they are constantly feeling pain. University of Texas researcher Jon Russell analyzed spinal fluid and found that fibro patients had substance P levels three times higher than normal.

Studies show that fibro patients tend to have elevated levels of nickel, mercury, cadmium, and lead, which inhibit production of serotonin and GABA. Hickey notes that it only takes about fifteen to twenty chelation treatments to reverse the ailment.

"Nobody knows what to do with these fibromyalgia patients," he says. "There are three approved medications, and none of them work. But chelation works beautifully. And most of these patients were sick for years. Fibromyalgia is my favorite disease because it gets better so easily with chelation."

Alzheimer's Disease

Perhaps no ailment is as heartbreaking as Alzheimer's disease and other forms of dementia, as a lifetime of memories are lost along with the ability to function independently. Alzheimer's not only destroys the lives of the afflicted but also their loved ones, who often serve as caretakers. Alzheimer's is draining emotionally, physically, and financially for all of those concerned. And it is affecting more and more of us every day: an estimated 5.8 million Americans as of this writing, with the number projected to sky-rocket to 13.8 million by 2050.

Despite hundreds of billions of dollars pumped into research over the past few decades, there remains no cure and no way to stop the progression of the disease. In fact, after all of that investment and time, and after intense study by some of the most brilliant scientists on Earth, we're still not even sure what causes Alzheimer's.

The message here is plain: Don't hold your breath waiting on a cure.

The only practical option is to try to prevent it, which offers much more hope. Reducing risk factors such as high blood pressure, high blood sugar, high cholesterol, obesity, smoking tobacco, and drinking alcohol can delay onset of the disease, potentially indefinitely. Chelation may also help, because brain tissue is very sensitive to heavy metals.

Wei Zheng, Ph.D., a professor of health sciences and toxicology at Purdue University, has been studying how heavy metals affect the brain for more than twenty years and is one of the world's foremost experts on the subject. He found that lead accumulation interferes with the way beta amyloid peptides are absorbed into cells, causing them to form amyloid plaque.

This accumulation is thought to disrupt communication between brain cells, which can result in the memory loss, motor dysfunction, and other types of cognitive decline that are the heartbreaking hallmarks of Alzheimer's disease.

"Beta amyloid is a naturally occurring protein in the brain that is water-soluble," explains Zheng. "When it interacts with the metal, it becomes not water-soluble and more prone to aggregation. That is how amyloid plaque is formed."

Zheng notes that the EPA considers any level of lead below 10 micrograms per deciliter to be okay.

"But academic study has already demonstrated that there is no safe level for lead concentration," he says. "If you find lead in the body, it is going to have some damaging effects."

He points out that the highest concentration of lead in the air occurred in the 1970s, before lead in gasoline started to be phased out as part of the Clean Air Act. Now, many people who were exposed back then are starting to reach prime Alzheimer's age.

"In the next ten years, we're going to see more Alzheimer's disease from the lead exposure," says Zheng. "So, if you have lead concentration in your blood, you have to get it out. Intravenous EDTA is quite effective."

Still, he doesn't recommend it for everyone.

"If you don't have any clinical symptoms, a better way may be to get a lot of exercise to keep the circulation active," Zheng suggests. "Drink a half cup of red wine every day too, because it stimulates microcirculation in the brain, and that is a way to get rid of the beta amyloid. Do brain exercises to challenge your mind, and amusing things to reduce stress."

Some people are at higher risk of Alzheimer's than others due to the ApoE gene, which produces a protein with 299 amino acids and comes in three varieties. ApoE4 is the one that increases risk of dementia up to twelve times, while ApoE2 protects against it. ApoE3 lies somewhere in the middle.

"The reason for that is ApoE2 has the amino acid cysteine at positions 112 and 159," says Hickey. "Cysteine is very negatively charged and is the body's natural chelator. It acts like a magnet, binding with the positively charged toxic metals that leak into the brain so they can be excreted.

"ApoE3, which has an average risk of dementia, only has one cysteine at 112, and arginine at 159, which doesn't have a negative charge. So, it has half the binding effect.

"ApoE4 has arginine at both of those positions, which means it has no negative charge. So, it can't bind metals, and they don't get eliminated."

Hickey recommends getting a genetic test and being more aggressively proactive if you have the ApoE4 variety.

"The trick is to catch it early, before the amyloid plaque builds up too much," he says. "Once people have Alzheimer's, it's tough to reverse."

Even so, TACT director Lamas noticed that EDTA chelation seemed to help the cognition of at least two of his diabetic patients in his peripheral artery disease pilot study. That inspired him to pursue a separate study, which quickly ran into a tough audience in the medical establishment.

"I put together a proposal and presented it to an Alzheimer's disease research center in Florida, and I essentially got laughed out of the committee room," says Lamas. "It's very frustrating."

Psoriasis

Psoriasis is an autoimmune disease, meaning the soldiers of the immune system get overstimulated and just start blasting away at everything, including healthy cells. That causes inflammation which, in the case of psoriasis, manifests in unsightly, red, scaly blemishes that can alter the trajectory of a person's whole life.

Consider Kevin Meany, who was literally never comfortable in his own skin.

"I had psoriasis for as long as I can remember," he says. "When I was in first grade, I was brutalized by my peers because I wasn't like them. I had it on my hands, arms, legs . . . everywhere. I tried every treatment known to man and nothing worked."

Kevin just learned to live with it, enduring not only the mental anguish from feeling different than others but also the endless discomfort of an inflamed epidermis. Still, he found a girl, got married, had kids, and wound up owning an advertising agency that's now part of a network he says grosses $1 billion a year. But he was always defined by his disease, at least until he met Hickey at a house party about fifteen years ago.

"Dr. Hickey told me what he was doing relative to holistic medicine and chelation, and I took it with a grain of salt," recalls Kevin. "But we ran into each other a few times after that, and he kept telling me to take a metal test because pollutants in the body can contribute to conditions like psoriasis and eczema. So, I finally took the test."

Turns out Kevin's mercury levels were "completely off the charts."

"I don't know how relevant it is, but as a kid, my friend had a jar of liquid mercury we used to play with a lot, and we had swordfights with florescent bulbs, getting white powder all over us when one broke," he says. "That was probably some pretty toxic stuff."

Hickey chelated Kevin with a combination of EDTA infusions and DMSA oral medications.

"He warned me it might get worse before it got better because some of the toxins are released through pores and irritate the skin," says Kevin. "I almost quit after getting four or five infusions, but I stuck with it. And by the tenth or twelfth treatment, my psoriasis had cleared up about 80 percent."

Now, psoriasis is basically a non-factor in Kevin's life.

"I pretty much don't have it," he says. "People who haven't seen me in years are surprised to see my skin look so great. Every once in a while, I get a little patch, but nothing much. If I go too long without a treatment, it starts coming back worse. So, I go to see Dr. Hickey, I get chelated and it goes away."

Kevin, who's now sixty-five years old, says he feels better than ever physically, and also feels great about himself.

"Having psoriasis had a huge impact on my life, particularly in my teenage years. And that changed my whole outlook," he says. "Being able to wear a pair of shorts or a short-sleeve shirt and not be self-conscious is an amazing experience for me."

Chelation helped another one of Hickey's patients with a different skin problem.

"About four years ago, I woke up with hives on my stomach and back," says Sheri Prudhomme. "I tried taking (the over-the-counter antihistamine) Benadryl, but it got progressively worse."

An allergist gave her a couple of medications, but the hives just kept coming.

"They were everywhere, first on my trunk, then moving up and down my legs, on my face, in my hair and ears, even in my privates," she confides.

Desperate, she went to the Mayo Clinic in Jacksonville, Florida. Among other things, she says they gave her a pill normally used for "major league depression, and after two days of taking it, I'd turned into a zombie." An IV steroid treatment seemed to help at first, but the relief only lasted a couple of days.

"All along, a friend had referred me to Dr. Hickey, but I was unsure about chelation and stayed with my allergist," she says. "I was on eighteen medications and one Xolair shot a month when I finally decided enough was enough. The hives were all over, and the medications seemed to be adding gasoline to the fire. I had weird, raised hives, some bigger than half-dollars. I felt terrible and was embarrassed to go out."

Hickey ran some tests and discovered that Sheri had high levels of heavy metals and a severe vitamin deficiency that he blamed on the medications.

"I got chelation, and it turned out to be the best day of my life," proclaims the fifty-three-year-old. "Dr. Hickey said it would take some time to work, but within two weeks I looked and felt like a different person."

She still gets chelation infusions about once a month and feels that the benefits are more than skin deep for her.

"I've got a lot more energy, and am much more clear-headed," she says. "Another crazy thing is the chelation got rid of the sunspots I had on my hands and shoulders. It's just amazing."

Macular Degeneration

Ophthalmologist Dr. Edward Kondrot first got interested in chelation when it relieved his uncle's chest pain. That piqued his curiosity about a therapy he'd always assumed to be quackery and a waste of money. Then he ran into Dr. Harold Behar, a fellow ophthalmologist he'd known from his days as a resident in Philadelphia. Kondrot remembered Behar as being "conservative" and was surprised to hear his old pal was using chelation in his practice.

"I'm getting good results," Behar told him. "It's turning macular degeneration patients around."

That encounter convinced Kondrot to start investigating the benefits of chelation. He joined ACAM, got certified in the administration of IV chelation, and began to use it in his own practice.

"I started doing a six-hour challenge test on my patients and discovered that a vast majority of those with serious eye problems, like macular degeneration, cataracts, and glaucoma, had heavy-metal loads that were off the chart," he says. "Just about every eye patient I treated had some improvement in his or her vision. It wasn't a cure in and of itself, but chelation therapy became an important part of my practice."

Chelation works on two levels for eye problems. First, it improves circulation in the tiny blood vessels that nourish the eyes. It also removes toxic metals that are particularly damaging to the lens and retinal tissue. Kondrot uses it in combination with other modalities, including microcurrent stimulation, syntonic light therapy, biofeedback, and homeopathy.

One of his patients was the late beer brewing magnate Bill Coors, who wrote the foreword for Kondrot's 1999 book, *Healing the Eye the Natural Way*. In it, he recalls how, in the mid-1980s, he was told by his ophthalmologist: "You have age-related macular degeneration. It is the leading cause of blindness in older people. We have no treatment for it. Come back and see me in three months."

Coors refused to accept that hopeless prognosis and turned to alternative therapies. Along with chelation, he took nutritional supplements, did all he could to bolster his immune system, and optimized his mental attitude.

"At this writing, I have sixteen more years of life expectancy," he says in the foreword. "I have every confidence that at the end of those years, I will see well enough to enjoy a gorgeous sunset and feast on the faces of those I love."

Coors surpassed his life expectancy, dying in 2018 at the ripe old age of 102. And his prophecy that he'd be able to see the beauty of nature and his loved ones till the end of his days came true.

IN THEIR OWN WORDS

I discovered I had breast cancer when I saw the lump protruding from my breast. I always knew if I ever got cancer, I would never go the conventional route to deal with it. I heard about Utopia Wellness in Florida and went down there. I got it in my head that I would be out of there in six weeks and be cancer-free. And I was. I worked very hard at healing myself. Dr. Garcia provides all the tools, and chelation is one of them. Although you need more than just getting heavy metals out of your body, I really believe that chelation is an important part of healing for most diseases. My body is healthier now, but the biggest changes were mental. I believe I brought cancer into my life because my life was so stressful and unhappy, and that was my only way out. I feel blessed to have had cancer because it made me take steps to change my life for the better.

Marion T., 57, Long Island, New York

CHAPTER 12

Chelation as Part of a Holistic Approach to Care

While chelation therapy is a vital tool in achieving optimal health, it should be just one part of a comprehensive strategy that is individualized for each person. The complexities of the human body are such that we generally need more than reducing toxic heavy-metal contamination to prevent or fight disease. Many of us have a deficiency of essential nutrients, and/or candida overgrowth, and/or thyroid dysfunction, and/or contamination by other toxins, and/or a number of other things. So, it's likely that you will need more than chelation to set you right.

"We do three things in treating a patient," says Dr. John Parks Trowbridge. "Number One is to find what is blocking you from getting better—such as toxic metals—and remove it. Number Two is to determine what you need to repair yourself—such as nutrients—and provide what is missing. The third thing is to turn on the switches to the healing processes—such as using hormone replacement or oxygen therapy—then step back and get out of the way. God built the system and knows how to make it work much better than we do."

Finding the Root Cause

If you're like most people, you go to your conventional family doctor for an annual exam, which usually includes a standard blood/urine panel measuring general levels of cholesterol, glucose, various types of blood cells, a smattering of vitamins and minerals, maybe a hormone or two, and other things. It offers the physician a peephole into your physicality, which may or may not set off alarms that something has gone wrong.

If you have high cholesterol, the doctor may talk to you about lifestyle changes but will likely write you a prescription for a statin because it's easier to take a pill than lose weight and get regular exercise. High blood sugar? Take some diabetes medication. High blood pressure? Take hypertension medication.

See a pattern here? Whatever the symptom, there is a drug to alleviate it. But alleviating symptoms doesn't fix the inherent problem. Rather than asking what drug can fix the symptom, you're better off asking what's going on in your body to cause things like high cholesterol or high blood pressure.

HIDDEN HEALTH PROBLEMS

Just as heavy-metal contamination can sabotage your health without you realizing it, there are some other insidious conditions that often fly under the radar. Here are some of the most common:

- **Mold:** If you have water stains in your home, school, or workplace, chances are you're being exposed to toxic mold spores. The spores have been linked to a variety of ailments, including chronic fatigue, autoimmune disorders, digestive problems, hormonal disruptions, breathing trouble, and neurological issues.

- **Parasites:** Protozoa parasites are single-cell organisms that can cause diarrhea and other digestive problems. If they breach the intestinal tract and enter the bloodstream, they can affect organs, including the heart and brain. Worm parasites, called helminths, also affect the intestinal tract, and their excrement can trigger inflammatory reactions throughout the body, resulting in a variety of symptoms.
- **Candida:** Overgrowth of this yeast crowds out good gut flora and releases toxins that can cause chronic fatigue, mood swings, digestive problems, sinus infections, brain fog, hormonal imbalances, allergies, headaches, and the list goes on.
- **Lyme disease:** Caused by tick-borne bacteria, Lyme disease is called The Great Imitator because symptoms can mirror other health woes, such as flu, arthritis, chronic fatigue, fibromyalgia, multiple sclerosis, and Alzheimer's. The telltale sign is a bull's-eye rash around the tick bite, but not every victim gets it.
- **Leaky gut:** Normally, intestinal tissue only lets small beneficial particles into the bloodstream, but malfunctions of gateways called intestinal tight junctions allow larger, potentially damaging things such as microbes and toxins to pass through. The body reacts by launching an inflammatory response, which can trigger a variety of ailments and symptoms.
- **Obstructive sleep apnea (OSA):** Snoring is not only annoying to a bedmate but also a sign of OSA, in which breathing stops repeatedly during the night. That will rob you of the regenerative processes that occur during deep sleep stages and can eventually contribute to serious health conditions, including hypertension, weight gain, type 2 diabetes, cardiac arrhythmias, stroke, congestive heart failure, and heart attack.

Trowbridge and his integrative brethren focus on finding the root cause of the problem and trying to fix it at the source. For example, remove toxic metals and you may not need the statins or hypertension meds. But you likely won't find the root cause(s) to a degenerative disease through the standard blood/urine panel.

"In my practice, we've evolved a set of tests designed to reveal key parameters related to progression of degenerative diseases," says Trowbridge. "In particular, that means monitoring the degree of inflammation chemistry."

Along with the heavy-metal challenge test described in Chapter 5 and heart diagnostics usually performed by cardiologists, the following are some of the tests Trowbridge and others employ:

- **Ferritin:** Increased blood levels of ferritin is a biomarker for iron overload, which is closely associated with atherosclerosis and various types of heart disease.

- **Protein Unstable Lesion Signature Test (PULS):** Most heart attacks are caused by ruptures of unstable plaque in coronary arteries. The unstable lesions leak unique proteins, which this test measures. It's a good indicator of overall heart health and risk for a cardiac event.

- **Zone 2 Cellular Inflammation:** This simple finger-stick blood test measures the levels of two key fatty acids in the blood: arachidonic acid (AA) an omega-6, and eicosapentaenoic acid (EPA), an omega-3. The ratio between them is a biomarker for cellular inflammation. The higher the level of cellular inflammation, the higher the risk of developing a chronic disease, and the faster the progression of it.

- **Homocysteine level:** High levels of homocysteine can contribute to arterial damage and blood clot formation. It is often due to a deficiency in vitamin B12 (folate).

- **Vitamin D:** It may come as a surprise that vitamin D is actually a hormone produced in the body with the help of sun exposure. It is a vital element in many biological functions, and chronic deficiency has been linked to an increasing number of degenerative diseases.

- **ANA and ESR:** Antinuclear antibody (ANA) and erythrocyte sedimentation rate (ESR) measured via blood tests can be an indication of inflammation and autoimmune issues.

- **Comprehensive Digestive Stool Analysis:** Biomarkers from this test offer a comprehensive look at the health of the gastrointestinal tract.

- **Sleep Oximetry Testing:** Using a simple finger probe, pulse and oxygen saturation can easily be determined, possibly signaling oxygen absorption problems during sleep. Low oxygen levels can contribute to many chronic problems, including high blood pressure, heart disease, stroke, arthritis, digestive disturbances, and cancer.

- **Biological Terrain Assessment (BTA):** This test uses blood, urine, and saliva to give an overall assessment of health. It can detect pH balance, resistivity (to help determine mineral deficiencies), as well as levels of antioxidants, digestive enzymes, and other biomarkers.

- **Autonomic Response Testing (ART):** A biofeedback assessment based on muscle tone, ART reveals hidden problems in the autonomic system that controls heartbeat, breathing, and other involuntary functions.

- **Computerized Regulation Thermography (CRT):** This diagnostic tool measures precise skin temperature fluctuations that can signal specific health problems. One German study found it much more effective in diagnosing breast cancer than mammography.

Other Therapies

Just as fine wine (or beer) pairs well with certain foods, chelation pairs well with some other therapies. They include:

- **Hyperbaric oxygen therapy:** Initially used for deep-sea divers who suffered decompression sickness—a.k.a., bends—hyperbaric oxygen chambers have become a staple in both conventional and alternative medicine for a variety of conditions. The chamber forces pure oxygen into the lungs, typically at three times the normal pressure. This allows highly oxygenated blood to reach damaged areas, speeding up recovery. In the conventional medical world, it is mainly used for non-healing wounds, some types of infections, and a few other specific problems.

  Alternative practitioners believe that the healing power of oxygen can help a wide range of conditions, including heart disease, cancer, and Alzheimer's. "Hyperbaric oxygen is one of the best things you can use when you're doing chelation therapy," says Dr. Carlos Garcia. "It basically acts like a pressure cooker, so the oxygen penetrates the organs. The more deeply the organs get penetrated with oxygen, the better they function."

- **Ozone therapy:** People may associate ozone with air pollution, but it actually is a natural cleansing agent for both the air and the body. The ozone molecule differs from oxygen by having three oxygen atoms instead of two, which gives it more energy to kill pathogens and heal damaged tissue. Therapeutic ozone is delivered in a variety of ways, including rectally or by injection, infusion, and even a type of dialysis. "Ozone and chelation therapy very much complement each other," says Dr. Robert Rowen, co-founder of the integrative RowenSu Clinic in Santa Rosa, California.

"Ozone gets more oxygen into the system and helps improve circulation and mitochondria function, and chelation helps to clear calcium out of the arteries and remove heavy metals. I do them on the same day because they're synergistic."

One patient Rowen says benefited from that synergy was the late ophthalmologist Dr. Gerald Foy. "He went from being almost crippled to digging fence posts on his property in a matter of weeks through ozone and chelation therapy," says Rowen. "He loved chelation. But I believe ozone is the stuff of the future. It will eclipse everything."

- **Microcurrent:** This technique uses a very low current of electricity at a specific frequency to stimulate tissue and speed up healing. Among other things, it is said to greatly increase the activity of adenosine triphosphate (ATP), which is basically the body's fuel. This creates more cellular energy. Integrative ophthalmologist Dr. Edward Kondrot finds that chelation is enhanced by microcurrent therapy in treating age-related macular degeneration. "I was introduced to microcurrent when I read that Sam Snead, the famous golfer, had a reversal of his macular degeneration using microcurrent," says Kondrot. "It is a way to improve blood flow and stimulate cellular activity. It can help mobilize heavy metals. It supports the kidney, liver, and lymphatic system during any type of chelation process. I made it part of my protocol with all the patients I was treating who had heavy-metal poisoning and chronic eye disease."

On a side note, while Kondrot was visiting Snead in Florida, the links legend offered to give him golf lessons. But after seeing the eye doctor's swing on the driving range, Snead told him: "Here is my advice. I want you to cut back on golf for a year, and then I want you to just give it up."

- **Holistic dentistry:** Silver fillings (amalgams) are about 50 percent mercury and have come under much scrutiny in recent years. While the American Dental Association, the FDA, and many other esteemed organizations insist they are safe, a growing number of other experts disagree. "Liquid mercury and mercury vapor are relatively non-reactive by themselves, which is why the dental people say, 'It's inert,'" notes microbiologist Anne Summers. "But everything is only inert until it comes in contact with the next strong catalyst, and there are some very strong catalyzing agents in the hearts of proteins."

  For example, the enzyme catalase transforms inert mercury into a very reactive ion. While no one disputes that mercury is a neurotoxin and can cause or contribute to neurological problems and other chronic diseases, they don't all agree whether or not the trace amounts of vapor exposure from fillings do any physiological harm. Most chelation practitioners believe that the cumulative impact over decades of filling degradation through chewing, brushing, and corrosion can indeed be very damaging. They often recommend that patients with amalgam fillings get them replaced with less toxic composite, porcelain, or metal substances.

  Be aware that the amalgam removal procedure itself can be dangerous, not only to the patient but even to the dentist and his staff. It takes special training and precautions to make sure the fix doesn't cause even more problems.

- **Nutritional supplements:** Because EDTA and other chelators remove some essential nutrients along with the toxic metals, it's highly recommended that all patients take a potent multivitamin/mineral. Dr. John Parks Trowbridge suggests extra doses of magnesium, to aid circulation, and EPA, an omega-3 fatty acid that is critical for reducing inflammation. He also suggests a full range of vitamin E supplements containing both tocotrienols and tocopherols.

Studies show that when they are taken together, they provide endothelial support to keep blood vessels healthy. Another beneficial supplement is nattokinase, an enzyme extracted from fermented soy beans that makes blood platelets "less sticky," thus reducing the risk of clot formation. The essential metal molybdenum is a vital part of chelation nutritional support. That's because a deficiency of it impairs sulfur-handling enzymes, which can spark adverse effects from chelation.

- **Lifestyle:** By now, you should know that chelation therapy is only part of the program when it comes to optimizing your health. All of the practitioners interviewed for this book do their best to educate their patients about how best to live a healthy lifestyle. It starts with eating right: opting for whole foods over the processed stuff, choosing organic to reduce exposure to pesticides and other toxins, limiting portion size, and going easy on the alcohol.

  Regular exercise is also important. You don't have to join a gym or run marathons. Vigorous walking is perhaps the easiest and most convenient way to increase blood circulation and reap other benefits of movement. Shoot for at least a half-hour every day. It's also good to do some resistance training, such as weights or calisthenics, to slow down the natural loss of muscle mass that comes with aging. Along with diet and exercise, you should try to reduce stress through deep breathing, meditation, and other methods; get between seven and eight hours of quality sleep a day; and maintain social connections.

- **Other things:** Depending on a patient's specific health woes and physiology, various other treatments may complement chelation. They include acupuncture, chiropractic, massage, detox cleanses, aromatherapy, reflexology, homeopathy, biofeedback, and bio-identical hormone replacement.

IN THEIR OWN WORDS

I had a problem with a small vein in my leg that got blocked up so badly I had to go every fourth month to get heparin (injections). Meanwhile, I had brown spots on my left leg and one turned into an ulcer. The doctors at the hospital told me there was a 75 percent chance they were going to have to amputate the leg, so I started going to see Dr. Trowbridge. He chelated me but it didn't do much until he gave me some nattokinase (an enzyme extracted from fermented soybeans). Everything healed up wonderfully, but I still had the brown spots. So, I got some chelation cream from the Internet and rubbed it on the spots, and now they're just about gone. Between the chelation infusions, nattokinase, and chelation cream, I'm back on my feet. I can tap dance, and I didn't need anyone to cut me open or put plastic (stents) in my veins.

Lee A., 71, Houston, Texas

CHAPTER 13

The Great Divide Between Conventional Medicine and Alternative Healing

Despite chelation's potential in combating a variety of health conditions, the therapy remains one of the most well-defined battlefields between two main factions of the medical community.

Just like the great political divide between Red and Blue America, there is a deep chasm separating medical care in this country. On one side is conventional medicine, and across the breach lies the camp of alternative medicine. Their differences are stark, and as in the political landscape, emotions often run high.

Alternative practitioners see their conventional counterparts as beholden to the pharmaceutical industry and pawns in the healthcare insurance juggernaut. Conventional docs contend that the alternative medicine universe is too lightly regulated and rife with unproven therapies that may not only be a waste of money to patients but also a risk to their health. To some degree, both sides are right, and wrong.

Some physicians have been trying to straddle the divide but, more and more, seem to be favoring the alternative side. Called integrative, complementary, or functional doctors, most of them practiced conventional medicine when they entered the profession, but they eventually became disenchanted with the focus on pharmaceuticals and procedures. They have broadened their scope to not only include many alternative therapies, but prioritize them.

"Our type of medicine simply involves trying to get into a person's body what it needs to heal, and get out of the body what is screwing up its healing," says Dr. Robert Rowen. "That's all there is to it."

Dr. John Parks Trowbridge adds: "The problem with conventional medical doctors is that they don't treat the mechanisms by which we get sick. Instead, they look at the pathological processes in which a drug can be applied. Drugs are stoppers. They don't make things work better. They stop certain things your body is doing on the inside."

Integrative physicians like Rowen, Trowbridge, and Dr. Tammy Born consider the primary tools of the conventional trade—drugs and surgeries—to be last resorts rather than first options. While these doctors are armed with the power to prescribe medications, they do so judiciously and as part of a broader holistic treatment plan.

"I still write prescriptions every day," says Born. "But if I need to give someone an antibiotic, I also give them probiotics and other things to protect their liver and gut from the negative side effects."

Perhaps the biggest difference is that integrative doctors are more focused on preventative care, because they feel that the best way to deal with a disease is to treat it before it fully emerges.

"Traditional medicine is a wait-and-see system," notes Born. "They wait until you get sick to treat you. There's no proactivity, no real sense of prevention beyond, 'Go and get your flu shot.' My son-in-law is in medical school, and they still don't teach nutrition, which is really the most basic of all preventative measures.

"That's the way it is, and nothing is going to change from the doctors. It's going to change from the patients, and it's up to us to educate them. We need to teach them to think proactively and understand that they have to take responsibility for their own health."

Another big difference between the two camps is the amount of time they typically spend with their patients. Often, hospitals and corporate clinics limit examinations to ten or fifteen minutes. It's something that neither doctors nor patients like, but seeing more patients means more money, and the bottom line has pretty much overtaken patient care as the most critical factor in the American healthcare system.

Conventional doctors also complain bitterly about the amount of "paperwork" they are forced to do to satisfy insurance companies and government regulations, including the widely detested electronic medical records (EMR). The administrative requirements can take up as much as half of a physician's workday, which translates into fewer patients getting less attention. It also contributes to a growing trend of doctor burnout.

In a *Newsmax* magazine article, Dr. Leif Dahleen, a forty-two-year-old anesthesiologist from Minnesota, says that "administrative hassles" were part of the reason he cut his working hours by 40 percent.

"Being burdened by the EMR and excessive paperwork adds to the stress of an already stressful job," he explains. "Doctors want to spend more time with their patients and have more autonomy in how they practice medicine."

But that's clearly not going to happen anytime soon, leaving both doctors and their patients frustrated. Most integrative doctors avoid those constraints by being independent entities.

That allows the doctors to spend a half-hour or more with each patient, giving them the kind of attention they're not likely to find in the conventional medicine world. But it comes at a high price because the integrative docs typically don't accept insurance, and care can easily cost thousands of out-of-pocket dollars over the course of a year.

"I do accept Medicare," says Born. "I don't want to not take care of old, poor people. Medicare won't pay for chelation, but it will pay for most of the lab work and some other things."

She does her best to keep prices down. In the tail end of 2019, each hour-and-a-half chelation treatment cost $95, or $1,900 for a series of twenty, which she often recommends to patients with high levels of heavy metals. Those rates are about as low as you'll find, with some practitioners charging double that, or even more.

Of course, most conventional physicians will say you might as well toss that money straight into the toilet, where the EDTA and those trace amounts of heavy metals wind up. You may recall renowned Cleveland Clinic cardiologist Dr. Steven Nissen declaring that chelation is part of a "quack approach" with no scientific evidence to support its purported benefits.

Yet not all scientific evidence accepted by the conventional medical community has exactly worked out as anticipated. For example, the revolutionary extended-release pain medication OxyContin was declared to be longer lasting than previous opioid medications after being studied in trials funded by the drug's manufacturer Purdue Pharma, which heavily marketed OxyContin to an embracing medical establishment.

"Scientific evidence amassed over more than 20 years, including more than a dozen controlled clinical studies, supports FDA's approval of 12-hour dosing for OxyContin," Purdue's chief medical officer, Dr. Gail Cawkwell, declared in a written statement to *The Los Angeles Times*.

Unfortunately, the painkiller's effects wore off hours sooner for a lot of people, leading to higher-dosage prescriptions. That helped spark an epidemic of addiction and overdoses that continues to rage across America. The impact has been nothing less than catastrophic. The government's CDC branded the drug and its ilk as a major cause for the shocking drop in life expectancy in the U.S. over the past three years.

Even studies not conducted by pharmaceutical companies suffer from reliability problems.

"The majority of papers that get published, even in serious journals, are pretty sloppy," says Stanford University professor of medicine John Ioannidis, who specializes in the study of scientific studies. "Across biomedical science and beyond, scientists do not get trained sufficiently on statistics and on methodology."

In an essay called "Why Most Published Research Findings Are False," Ioannidis adds: "For many current scientific fields, claimed research findings may often be simply accurate measures of the prevailing bias."

While physicians like Nissen tend to readily accept data from studies that support their own beliefs, in chelation's case they are quick to discount not only the "gold-standard" TACT study but also mountains of observational and clinical evidence accumulated over decades that supports chelation's many benefits, especially with cardiovascular issues.

The best of both worlds would be if the conventional and alternative camps could start working together better, using all of the resources available to fight the common enemy of disease. Occasionally, it already happens. Dr. Trowbridge tells this story:

"About twenty years ago, a downtown Houston cardiologist, who had referred me an occasional patient interested in chelation, sent me a gentleman in his late seventies. He needed bypass surgery and repair of heart muscle damage, but his heart and general physical condition were such that the surgeons felt an operation posed too high a risk. I explained how chelation might help, and the man turned out to be a compliant, even enthusiastic, patient. After some four-dozen treatments, he returned to his cardiologist for follow-up.

"Soon thereafter, I received an unexpected letter from his doctor. He expressed his appreciation for my care, because it helped the patient become eligible for the surgery he needed. He tolerated the procedures well and made an excellent recovery.

"Rather than 'competing' treatment programs, this showed that physicians with different technologies can, indeed, work together to provide the best outcome for patients."

Sadly, stories like that are more of an exception than the rule. Yet the explosion in this country of integrative MDs, who do try to provide patients with the best of both worlds, offers hope for a future of unity in the battle against an increasing array of medical conditions.

Family Affair

One thing of which there's little doubt to me is that the physicians who offer chelation therapy believe it works, evidenced by the fact that most of them who were interviewed for this book undergo the therapy themselves. Dr. Robert Battle, who runs the Comprehensive Health Center in Houston, Texas, credits doing regular sequences of chelation since 1982 for helping him to beat a genetic predisposition.

"I'm eighty-six years old and I have a strong family history of cardiovascular disease," says Battle. "Last November, I experienced some chest pain, so I got checked out by a cardiologist I sometimes refer patients to. He put me in the hospital overnight and did enzyme studies, EKGs, an echo(cardiogram) and an angio(gram). He said, 'Bob, you have the heart of a thirty-year-old. What are you doing here?'

"I had to confess that I'd had two eggs fried over easy and some buttered toast about an hour before Mass, and that it was probably just my gall bladder acting up because of the grease I had in that meal."

Dr. Trowbridge, who has lectured extensively about chelation and has been cited as a mentor for several of the practitioners I interviewed, says doctors have to "walk the talk."

"Since first offering chelation to my patients in 1983, I've personally enjoyed 580 IVs to enhance the nourishment of all of my organs," he says. "And I expect them to continue functioning delightfully for many years."

Dr. Born chelates herself, as well as her eighty-five-year-old father, Wesley Geurkink, a retired truck driver who boasts that he's never been admitted to a hospital in his life. But about thirty years ago, he noticed a strange sensation in the area of his jaw and was getting more out of breath than usual doing things like climbing stairs. His daughter checked him out, and a Doppler ultrasound test revealed some blockage in his carotid arteries.

"I did about fifteen chelation treatments, had another Doppler, and it showed no blockage at all," he says. "I continue to do it at least once a month, and I feel great."

Wesley is still very active, traveling with his second wife Sandi to Arizona in the winter, and in the summer he visits relatives in northern Minnesota, where he likes to fish. When in Michigan, he hangs out at his daughter's clinic on occasion, doing some handyman work because he likes to keep busy and help out.

"I don't know why it's taking so long to catch on," he says about chelation. "When you're here, you always hear people talking about how it's helped their health so much."

The Born Clinic's office manager, Elaine Fedewa, arranged to have her father Harold Zoll get chelation treatments. He was a heavy equipment mechanic most of his life, breathing in a lot of diesel exhaust, welding fumes, and even asbestos dust from brake linings. It didn't seem to affect his health much, but about twenty-five years ago, he lost vision in one eye and an ophthalmologist detected circulatory blockage.

"Elaine told me I needed to see Dr. Born and get some chelation," he recalls. "After four treatments my vision came back, and when I went to see the ophthalmologist, he said the blockage was gone."

Harold, now a robust ninety-five, eventually did fifty chelation treatments to reduce his heavy-metal load, then followed it up with the recommended once-a-month maintenance.

"Two years ago, I had some shortness of breath, and I went to a specialist in Lansing to check out my heart," he says. "He did an angiogram and said my (coronary) arteries were in better shape than his."

Truth is, everyone feels like family at the Born Clinic. It's an atmosphere created and maintained by Tammy Born, who knows that nurturing is an important part of the healing process.

When Michael Kanis arrives for his monthly infusion, he's greeted with a big hug from head IV nurse Liza Ewing before she hooks him up to the EDTA drip.

"The ladies who do this—I just love them," Michael says as he settles into one of the plush leather recliners for his chelation session. He's got a family history of heart disease and stroke, and ten years ago he suffered heart attack symptoms while on a business trip in Indiana.

"I thought I was going to pass out and pulled off the road at the first exit, and there was St. Mary Hospital, which has a full-blown heart center," says Michael, now fifty-eight.

Doctors at St. Mary determined that he was having a heart "incident," but not an attack, and suggested he see a cardiologist. Instead, he went to see Dr. Born, who had started treating his parents decades ago and serves as his family physician. She ran some tests and found that the femoral arteries in his legs had 70-plus percent blockage, while the carotids in his neck were 40 percent blocked. She prescribed chelation. He underwent two rounds of twenty treatments, which eliminated the tightness in his chest and other symptoms, and he has been doing monthly maintenance ever since.

"A year ago, I had an ultrasound for an unrelated issue, and my carotids had zero percent blockage," he says. "They didn't check my femoral arteries, but I'm sure they're clear because of the way I feel.

"I know my family history. I know how much my arteries were blocked. And I can honestly say that Tammy Born saved my life."

Michael used to do logistics for a Fortune 500 company but now runs his own small business distributing decorative stone for both residential and commercial properties. The dad of four and his wife Tina endured every parent's worst nightmare when their youngest daughter Caroline, whom they called "Peaches," was diagnosed with a very aggressive brainstem cancer. After she died at age nine, he and Tina launched a non-profit foundation called Caroline's PEACH, which stands for Philanthropic Endowment Advancing Children's Health, and is dedicated to making sick kids well.

"In Caroline's final days at our house, she needed IVs for nourishment, and Liza, the nurse here, traveled all the way there, forty-six miles and back, to do it," says Michael, the pain of his daughter's passing and the blessing of a good-hearted nurse combining to bring a tear to his eye. "After she died, the group at the

Born Clinic put together an Apple photo album of her that's now one of the most precious things we own. That's just so above and beyond. You're more than cared for here; you're loved. And you can't buy that."

IN THEIR OWN WORDS

In 2001, I was diagnosed with abdominal cancer, but it took them two years to figure out it was really metastasized lung cancer. I had chemo, radiation, and lung surgery, and the doctors said that if I survived all of that I still only had a one in five chance to live five years. Meanwhile, I developed a bad case of shingles and had pain 24/7. Dr. Trowbridge gave me chelation, some other treatments and supplements, and that cut my pain by about 80 percent. The pain is gradually leaving, and I expect it to leave completely. Six months ago, I called three out of four of my cancer doctors and left messages for them that I was still alive. I haven't heard a word from any of them. They're not even interested to know what I've done to live this long. I was in a bad hole and now I'm feeling so well, I don't know where the top is. That's a good problem to have.

Ida B.,* 73, Houston, Texas

*Pseudonym used by request.

CHAPTER 14

Starting Your Chelation and Finding Your Doctor

How to Find a Chelation Practitioner

The most comprehensive resource is the Chelation Physician Registry found on the chelation.me website. In the registry, which is associated with the International College of Integrative Medicine (ICIM), you will find each physician's name, address, and telephone number. Many of the entries also include email address, website, and a short bio. You can get a list of practitioners in the U.S. and Canada, or narrow it down to those in individual states.

http://chelation.me/chelation-physician-registry/

The American College for Advancement in Medicine (ACAM) website has a "Find a Practitioner Near You" listing. Just fill in your zip code, the mileage you are willing to travel, and click to get the names and contact information for practitioners certified by the ACAM.

https://www.acam.org/search/custom.asp?id=1758

Questions to Ask Your Practitioner

Are you licensed to prescribe chelation drugs?

The drugs used in chelation can only be prescribed by a medical doctor (MD), doctor of osteopathy (DO), dentist (DDS), and certified nurse practitioner (NP). Any other practitioner, including doctor of chiropractic (DC) and doctor of naturopathy (DN), would have to have the drug prescribed by someone with the aforementioned degrees.

Are you certified in chelation therapy? Where did you get your training?

Chelation is very safe when the accepted protocols are followed. To minimize risk, choose a practitioner who has been trained by either the American College for Advancement in Medicine or the International College of Integrative Medicine, both of which follow the protocol used in the TACT studies. Currently, the ACAM is the only certifying agency.

How long have you been performing chelation therapy? How many chelation patients have you treated?

Experience is a great teacher, and the more your practitioner has, the better.

Is a doctor physically present in the office when chelation treatments are administered? If not, who is responsible for managing any patient problems that might arise?

Some clinics may have medical doctors who prescribe the drugs but are often not present when the infusions are administered. Make sure someone qualified is always present to deal with anything unexpected.

How much do you charge? What does this include?

EDTA infusions run about $100 a pop and up. Costs typically range between $150 and $200. But some of those prices may be for the infusion alone, or they may include a consultation with the doctor, vitamin and mineral supplements, and other services or products. Some clinics offer package deals. Don't be shy about asking about costs up front. Some practitioners may offer a discount to needy patients.

Will private insurance or Medicare cover any of the costs associated with the chelation therapy?

Typically, neither private insurance nor Medicare will cover the costs of chelation therapy. But they may cover some costs of the lab tests, drugs, and complementary therapies. Ask the practitioner what will be involved, then speak with your insurance carrier to find out if you qualify for coverage for any of those aspects. One phone call could wind up saving you money.

Which chelating drugs will benefit my condition and why?

While infused disodium EDTA is the most common drug used by practitioners, several other drugs are also used, depending on what metals you harbor and other needs. The practitioner should be able to give you very specific reasons for prescribing any drug.

How many treatments are usually advised for someone with my condition?

Chelation is not a one-shot deal. Typically, practitioners will start with ten to twenty infusions. Dr. Lamas used forty in TACT 1 and 2. The sicker you are, the more infusions you're likely to need. Some patients require a hundred or more. It won't hurt to get an idea ahead of time so you will know how to budget your money and time.

Who produces the chelation drugs you use?

EDTA solutions and many other chelators are produced by compounding pharmacies. Your practitioner should know where they come from and when they were produced, as well as be able to vouch for their quality.

What are the ingredients of the chelation solution?

Once again, good doctors know exactly what they are giving their patients.

Concerning EDTA infusions, do you use the 3-gram or 1.5-gram version?

Both quantities appear to get similar results, but the 1.5-gram version takes half the time to infuse.

What other therapies do you recommend to complement chelation?

The answer to this question will likely be different for different patients. Chelation is just one tool in achieving good health, and you may require other therapies. Every chelation patient should at least get vitamin and mineral supplementation, because chelators can deplete some of these essential nutrients.

What kind of reactions or other problems should I be aware of?

Although chelation is generally safe, adverse reactions do occasionally occur. Be sure you know what to look for.

What should I read in order to really understand chelation therapy treatments?

The more you know about your condition and treatments, the better. Your doctor should be happy to help educate you.

Other Resources

The American Council for Advancement in Medicine. Chelation's greatest institutional champion, the ACAM website offers a comprehensive listing of articles and studies about the therapy, along with videos of patient experiences.

https://www.acam.org

Health Choices Now. The website of leading chelation practitioner Dr. John Parks Trowbridge offers a trove of articles and testimonials.

https://healthchoicesnow.com/treatments/chelation-therapy -detox

"Effect of Disodium EDTA Chelation Regimen on Cardiovascular Events in Patients with Previous Myocardial Infarction: The TACT Randomized Trial." The TACT 1 study article that appeared in the *Journal of the American Medical Association (JAMA)* in March 2013.

https://jamanetwork.com/journals/jama/fullarticle/1672238

A Textbook on EDTA Chelation Therapy. Edited by Elmer M. Cranton, M.D.; Hampton Roads Publishing Company; 2001. An anthology of chelation therapy studies with a foreword by the late Nobel Prize Laureate Linus Pauling.

The Scientific Basis of EDTA Chelation Therapy. Written by Bruce W. Halstead, M.D. and Theodore C. Rozema, M.D.; TRC Publishing; 1997. A detailed look at the physiological effects of chelation explains the science behind the therapy.

The Chelation Way: The Complete Book of Chelation Therapy. Written by Morton Walker, M.D.; Avery Publishing Group, Inc.; 1990. The podiatrist-turned–medical journalist describes the promise of chelation therapy, exemplified by several patient histories.

A Final Note

The story of chelation is as much a tale about ideology as anything else. For the conventional medicine crowd, chelation therapy seems to challenge their very belief system, in which a primary tenet is that good medicine can only emerge from well-established scientific method. For the most part, that leaves out traditional healing techniques that have been practiced around the world, often for thousands of years, as well as many alternative therapies that seem to help a lot of people but don't have the science to support their safety and efficacy.

While I respect science, the scientific methods practiced today have their shortcomings. The problem is that there really are no completely reliable data when it comes to medicine. Every scientific study is flawed to some degree, most notably the many that are funded by the pharmaceutical industry and are rife with conflicts of interest. Dr. Lamas' TACT 1 wasn't perfect, but it was probably less money-tainted than many and was overseen by people with impeccable credentials and reputations.

The truth is you don't need studies to get a good indication of whether or not a treatment works. Just talk to the patients. I interviewed dozens of chelation patients, and almost every one of them raved about how the therapy helped their health. Several of them even claimed it saved their lives. And most offered stories about others they've seen improve from a variety of degenerative diseases. They might not be doctors or scientists, but they know what has worked for them. And when you talk to enough of them, the aggregation of personal experience is likely to be as reliable as potentially accurate data amassed under controlled settings.

When critics can't argue with the substance, such as chelation relieving chest pain in heart patients or reversing gangrene in diabetics, they attack the process. One example is Lamas' TACT 1 study. Put anything under a microscope, and you will see flaws. Looking at the big picture, I see patients who are healed, or healing. They are also the most devoted patients I've ever encountered. They love their doctors not only because they believe the practitioners have helped their health—often when conventional medicine failed—but also because they feel their doctors love them.

Lamas comes from the conventional medical world and stresses that he is a scientist, not a chelation practitioner. He launched TACT 1 thinking he was going to prove that chelation was a waste of time and money. Yet his experiences studying the therapy and dealing with its practitioners have changed that belief and softened his views about alternative medicine.

"You get to know these people, have a few dinners and glasses of wine with them, hear about their kids, and then they tell you about their patients, and you don't think they are pulling your leg," he says. "It happens again and again, and even though you thought that chelation didn't do anything, a little doubt starts creeping in, and you think, 'What if there's something here?'"

Now, Lamas not only sees potential in chelation therapy but believes some of the other alternative medicine modalities may have merit.

"It makes you wonder what else is out there," he says.

After forty years of being a journalist, I find that the best information comes from people with firsthand knowledge and nothing to gain by lying. And in this case, I've heard the same story over and over again from the patients who have personally experienced the healing powers of chelation. The bottom line is well summed up by the words of heart disease patient Eugene Wisenbaker:

"Without chelation, I wouldn't be here today. I can say that for a fact."

Chelation
for Heart Disease

Chauncey W. Crandall IV, M.D., F.A.C.C.

As a cardiologist, I've seen chelation help my patients, although I must admit that I was initially surprised by this.

As a man of science, I was at first skeptical. I knew about chelation of course, and its usage that dates back to World War II, where it was used as an antidote against arsenic-based poison gas for sailors who had been exposed to lead-based paint on ships. Today, it is used to treat heavy metal poisoning, and this is the only usage for which it is approved.

I also knew that it was a popular alternative health treatment for several purposes, including coronary heart disease, but I am trained in the treatments of Western medicine that are evidence-based, which means they have been proven through clinical research to work.

I also knew that chelation was a popular alternative health treatment, but I tend to steer clear of treatments that do not have a solid track record of published studies behind them.

On the other hand, I was also trained as an anthropologist, doing field work in the jungles of Africa, and today, in addition to my cardiology practice in Florida, I spend my vacation time doing missionary work around the world, often in developing countries whose medical systems are looked down upon by my colleagues. I had seen them work, though, so I have a deep respect for them.

What changed my mind was, of course, was the Trial to Assess Chelation, or TACT study, that you've read about in this book. But I wanted to point out the things that impressed me, a veteran cardiologist whose practiced goes back four decades.

First, it really was a major study, conducted on 134 sites across the U.S. and Canada. Second, the sponsors were impressive: The National Institutes of Health's National Heart, Lung, and Blood Institute (NHLBI) and National Center for Complementary and Alternative Medicine (NCCAM), were impressive.

And, also very important, the study was "double blinded." A double-blinded study means that neither the doctors or the patients knew which whether the treatment was real or a sham, a method referred to as the "gold standard," of testing because it weeds out unconscious bias.

The initial results on these 1,708 heart attack survivors showed that it worked and achieved a modest benefit. But it was a finding within the subgroup of patients with diabetes that really blew me away.

People with diabetes are at high risk for heart attack, and there is little available to help. But this study showed that chelation reduced risk for diabetics by 39 percent and the risk reduction in people with a previous heart attack was 37 percent reduction in risk. This was an important finding.

I was also impressed that to see a similar finding in a follow-up study that was presented at the American Heart Association's 2013 Scientific Sessions. This study looked at 95 patients with diabetes and showed they had a 15 percent decrease in subsequent cardiac problems as compared to those who received the sham treatment. They found no such improvement in patients without diabetes. Also, in a more recent study, the researchers found that heart attack survivors who received oral high-dose vitamins along with chelation therapy reduced the risk of future cardiovascular problems by 26 percent. The results were even better for heart attack survivors with diabetes. In their case, the benefits of the combo therapy were even greater—51 percent— the researchers said.

I'm thinking in particular of one of my patients, Jim, who is a 70-year-old man with advanced heart disease. He is also a diabetic, and has suffered greatly from complications of that disease.

The complications of diabetes are deadly to the heart, and Jim already had undergone cardiac bypass surgery as well as stenting. But this metabolic disease also wreaks havoc on the rest of the body as well, and so Jim not only had heart problems, but he had severe peripheral vascular disease as well, which means that his circulation in his legs was diminished. In addition, he also suffered from a foot so ulcerated and impossible to heal that the vascular surgeon was recommending amputation as the last resort.

Sadly, this is not an uncommon occurrence in people with longstanding, severe diabetes, and Jim was understandably panicked. He had served in the Vietnam War and had seen his fellow soldiers suffer such fates. "Please, Dr. Crandall, isn't there anything else that can be done?" Jim implored me.

That's when I decided to recommend chelation. After 30 infusions, Jim's foot had improved to the point where amputation was no longer viewed as needed.

In addition to people with complications from diabetes like Jim, I also am inclined to recommend chelation to people who have inoperable heart disease, especially in the face of severe symptoms.

For most of my patients, I generally recommend conventional treatments. But for some patients with severe heart disease whose conditions do not respond to these methods, chelation may do the trick.

Chauncey W. Crandall IV, M.D., F.A.C.C., is Director of Preventive Medicine at the renowned Palm Beach Cardiovascular Clinic and Chief of Interventional Cardiology at Good Samaritan Medical Center in Palm Beach, Florida. He is also the editor of the popular medical newsletter, *Dr. Crandall's Heart Health Report.* Dr. Crandall 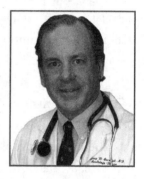 received his post-graduate training at Yale University School of Medicine, where he also completed three years of research in the Cardiovascular Surgery Division. In his over 25-year career, Dr. Crandall has performed over 40,000 heart procedures. He regularly lectures nationally and internationally on preventive cardiology, cardiology healthcare of the elderly, healing, interventional cardiology, and heart transplantation. Dr. Crandall has been heralded for his values and message of hope to all his heart patients.

Acknowledgments

No one can write a book like *The Chelation Revolution* in a vacuum, and I am deeply grateful to the many people who helped in one way or another. First and foremost is Chris Ruddy. Thanks to David Perel for recommending me for the job. I also appreciate the patience and fine work of Humanix Books publisher Mary Glenn and her team, who have turned my words into a beautifully crafted product.

This book would have been impossible for me to write without the help of the participating chelation practitioners and their patients, who openly shared with me their resources and experiences. Two in particular went above and beyond. Dr. Tammy Born invited me to her clinic in Grand Rapids, Michigan, so I could talk to patients and staff and even experience chelation therapy myself. And Dr. John Parks Trowbridge, who practices in Humble, Texas, not only was a veritable font of information about chelation but also offered me endless encouragement and was kind enough to proofread my manuscript for accuracy.

To my wife Nora, who always has my back. I am blessed to have such a positive influence in my life.

I'd like to offer a special thanks to my brother Rick, a cardiologist who set aside his skepticism about chelation to fully support my efforts. Most critically, he paved the way for me to connect with his colleague, TACT study director Dr. Tony Lamas. Along with being my brother, Rick is also the best friend anyone could ever have and a great doctor in his own right.

Of course, no one deserves more thanks than Dr. Lamas. He not only carved out time from his busy schedule to enlighten me about chelation through several lengthy phone interviews, but he also showed both courage and integrity in pursuing studies on chelation therapy. He continues to risk his sterling reputation as a physician and researcher to do the right thing, and his efforts have the potential to positively impact countless lives in the future.

Finally, I must not forget to thank you, the reader. Although writing this book was a rewarding experience in itself, it's far more rewarding to share it with others.

Index

AA (arachidonic acid), 144
ACAM (American College for
    Advancement in Medicine),
    35, 56, 161, 165
acam.org website, 165
acupuncture, 150
acute tubular necrosis, 57
addiction, 155
adenosine triphosphate (ATP), 50,
    147
advanced glycation end products
    (AGEs), 90
AGEs (advanced glycation end
    products), 90
AHA (American Heart
    Association), 3
ALA (alpha-lipoic acid), 66
alcohol, 149
alpha-lipoic acid (ALA), 66
alternative medicine
    cases/trials against, 14–15, 38,
        39
    vs. conventional medicine,
        151–154
    Lamas on, 7, 8
    negativity towards, 14, 17–18,
        37–40
    overview, 151–152
    Quackbusters and, 39

aluminum, 41, 51, 68–69, 71
Alzheimer's disease. *See also*
    cognition
    aluminum and, 51, 71
    arsenic in drinking water and,
        50
    chelation therapy and, 132–135
    lead and, 133
AMA (American Medical
    Association), 3, 38, 40
AMA Scientific Sessions, 80
amalgam fillings, 46–48, 57, 64,
    148
American College for
    Advancement in Medicine
    (ACAM), 35, 56, 161, 165
American College for
    Advancement of Medicine
    (ACAM), 12
American Heart Association
    (AHA), 3
American Institute of Medical
    Preventics, 12, 35
American Medical Association. *See*
    AMA
amputations, 13, 37, 107–110
amyloid plaque, 133, 134
ANA (antinuclear antibody), 144
anemia, 51, 126

heavy metals and, 73–86,
   100–101
iron and, 68–69
Lamas on, 16
lead and, 98–100
lifestyle changes, 26
pharmaceutical drugs, 82
plaque buildup, 76
stents, 78–81, 100–101
Trowbridge on, 89, 157
"widow-maker," 26, 94
Willix on, 81, 91
heavy metal challenge test, 60,
   64–65, 138, 144
heavy metal hypothesis, 91, 100
heavy metal toxicity, 1, 2
heavy metals
   affect on health, 42–44, 90–91
   aluminum, 41, 51, 68–69, 71
   Alzheimer's disease and,
      132–135
   arsenic, 49–50
   Born on, 43–44, 49, 103
   cadmium. *See* cadmium
   chromium, 52
   conditions associated with,
      128–129
   considerations, 32, 55
   diabetes and, 111
   fibromyalgia and, 131–132
   heart disease and, 73–86,
      100–101
   intestinal problems, 28
   iron, 51–52, 68–69
   Lamas on, 43–46, 98–100
   lead. *See* lead
   mercury. *See mercury entries*
   overview, 41–44
   post-partum depression and,
      129–130
   psoriasis and, 135–137
   PTSD and, 130–131
   reducing exposure to, 57
   removal of, 91
   sources of, 41–43
   Trowbridge on, 144

heavy-metal detoxication, 36
hemoglobin, 51
Henderson, Bill, 115
heparin, 70
Hickey, Joe, 66, 125–137
histone proteins, 99
hives, 136–137
Hochman, Judith, 80
holistic care, 141–150
   candida, 143
   finding root causes, 142–145
   holistic dentistry, 148
   hyperbaric oxygen therapy, 146
   leaky gut, 143
   lifestyle changes, 98, 149–150
   Lyme disease, 143
   microcurrent therapy, 147–148
   mold, 142
   nutritional supplements,
      148–149
   obstructive sleep apnea, 143
   other treatments, 150
   overview, 141
   ozone therapy, 146–147
   parasites, 143
holistic dentistry, 148
homeopathy, 150
homocysteine level, 144
hydrochloride, 70
Hyman, Mark, 48
hyperbaric oxygen therapy, 109, 146

IBCMT (International Board of
   Clinical Metal Toxicology),
   56
ICIM (International College of
   Integrative Medicine), 56,
   161, 162
immune system, 45
inflammation, 90, 144
infused EDTA, 36, 63
insurance companies, 95–96
insurance coverage, 19, 95–96, 154,
   163
integrative doctors, 151–152, 153,
   156

sleep oximetry testing, 145
smoke, cigarette, 48, 49
Snead, Sam, 147–148
sodium bicarbonate, 70
soft drinks, 61
sperm counts, low, 45
spinal cord, 131
statins, 82, 83
statistics, 155
stenosis, 94
stent procedures, 78–81, 100–101
stomach cancer, 28
stool analysis, 145
stress, 81, 149–150
studies/trials, 35–36
    CABG studies, 94
    cancer studies, 119
    cardiovascular studies, 35–36,
      37–38
    considerations, 3
    COURAGE study, 79
    early, 3, 12–13
    EDTA chelation clinical trials,
      36–37
    ISCHEMIA study, 80, 82
    JUPITER trial, 83–84
    peripheral artery disease, 59,
      107–110, 113–114
    placebo-controlled studies, 3
    Scandinavian, 13
    TACT. See TACT entries
substance P, 131
succimer, 64
Summers, Anne, 47, 148
supplements, 8, 9, 10, 148–149
suppositories, EDTA, 63

TACT (Trial to Access Chelation
    Therapy)
    attacks from medical community,
      13–18
    challenges, 7–9
    considerations, 4
    diabetes sub-group, 9, 16, 19
    findings, 9, 15–18
    importance of, 7, 38

    infusion ingredients used in,
      69–70
    Lamas on, 7
    landmark study, 7–20
    number of EDTA infusions,
      9, 10
    origin of, 3–4
    participants, 9, 10
    purpose, 9
    results, 9, 15–20
    scope, 9
    standards, 9
    suspension of, 14–15
    Willix on, 8
TACT 1 study, 92–94, 99
TACT 2 study, 18–19, 20, 100
TACT 3a study, 19, 111–114
T-cells, 45
thiamine, 70
thimerosal, 47
tobacco smoke, 48, 49
tooth fillings, 46–48, 57, 64, 148
Topol, Eric, 18
toxins. See heavy metals; poisons
traditional medicine. See conven-
    tional medicine
Trial to Access Chelation Therapy.
    See TACT
trials. See studies/trials
Trowbridge, John Parks
    on chelation infusion recipe,
      69–70
    on conventional medicine,
      73–74, 152
    on DMPS, 64
    early experience with chelation,
      74–75
    on heart disease, 89, 157
    on heavy metals, 144
    holistic approach to care,
      141–150
    on nutritional supplements,
      149
    on personal chelation, 157
    practitioner profile, 67
tubular necrosis, 57

About the Author

Gary Greenberg is an award-winning journalist who has primarily worked as a newspaper reporter, columnist, and editor. He now owns the freelance writing service SuperWriter, Inc. and specializes in natural and alternative health stories. He's written hundreds of articles that have appeared in a variety of regional and national publications, including *Newsmax*, *AARP*, and *Life Extension* magazines. During his journalism career, Gary spent thirteen years as a staff writer/editor for AMI, Inc., publishers of the *National Enquirer* and other tabloids.

Gary lives in Boca Raton, Florida, with his wife Nora. They have a grown son, Glen, as well as rescue dog Roxanne, birds Baba and Olaf, turtles Stella and Dottie, and bearded dragon lizard Klaus.

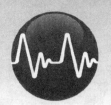

Simple **Heart Test**

Powered by Newsmaxhealth.com

FACT:

▸ Nearly half of those who die from heart attacks each year never showed prior symptoms of heart disease.

▸ If you suffer cardiac arrest outside of a hospital, you have just a 7% chance of survival.

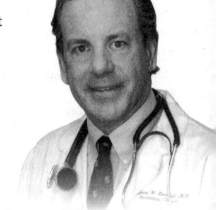

Don't be caught off guard. Know your risk now.

TAKE THE TEST NOW ...

Renowned cardiologist **Dr. Chauncey Crandall** has partnered with **Newsmaxhealth.com** to create a simple, easy-to-complete, online test that will help you understand your heart attack risk factors. Dr. Crandall is the author of the #1 best-seller *The Simple Heart Cure: The 90-Day Program to Stop and Reverse Heart Disease.*

Take Dr. Crandall's Simple Heart Test — it takes just 2 minutes or less to complete — it could save your life!

Discover your risk now.

- Where you score on our unique heart disease risk scale
- Which of your lifestyle habits really protect your heart
- The true role your height and weight play in heart attack risk
- Little-known conditions that impact heart health
- Plus much more!

SimpleHeartTest.com/Metal

Improve Memory and Sharpen Your Mind

Misplacing your keys, forgetting someone's name at a party, or coming home from the market without the most important item — these are just some of the many common memory slips we all experience from time to time.

Most of us laugh about these occasional memory slips, but for some, it's no joke. Are these signs of dementia, or worse, Alzheimer's? Dr. Garry Small will help dissuade those fears and teach you practical strategies and exercises to sharpen your mind in his breakthrough book, *2 Weeks To A Younger Brain*.

This book will show that it only takes two weeks to form new habits that bolster cognitive abilities and help stave off or even reverse brain aging.

If you commit only 14 days to *2 Weeks To A Younger Brain*, you will reap noticeable results. During that brief period, you will have learned the secrets of keeping your brain young for the rest of your life.

Claim Your FREE OFFER Now!

Claim your **FREE** copy of *2 Weeks To A Younger Brain* — a $19.99 value — today with this special offer. Just cover $4.95 for shipping & handling.

Plus, you will receive a 3-month risk-free trial subscription to *Dr. Gary Small's Mind Health Report*. Renowned brain expert and psychiatrist Gary Small, M.D., fills every issue of *Mind Health Report* with the latest advancements and breakthrough techniques for improving & enhancing your memory, brain health, and longevity. **That's a $29 value, yours FREE!**

Natural 'Super Citrus' Breakthrough Gently Supports Crucial Body Detoxification

Right this very minute, your body is under attack. Even if you eat well and enjoy a healthy lifestyle . . .

Your body faces constant challenges from an accumulation of environmental chemicals, heavy metals, additives, and other toxins.

What's worse, these toxins are everywhere.

They are in your food, your air, and the water you drink and bathe in. **Worst of all, they are in YOU.** It's easy to see that when your body is overloaded with toxins.

Some toxins damage cellular DNA. Others disrupt normal hormone function — or even the performance of your immune system.

EVERTO Supports Cellular Health and Gentle Detoxification

EVERTO is a unique patented formula containing Modified Citrus Pectin (MCP).

MCP supports your cells by blocking a rogue protein.

Regular, unmodified citrus pectin has molecules too large for the body to absorb.

So scientists devised a breakthrough proprietary enzymatic and pH process. This modifies pectin to ensure its molecules are more easily absorbed by the body.

So why would they go through all this trouble? Well, this brings us to something called galectin-3.

In excess amounts, this Velcro-like protein encourages certain unhealthy cells to clump together and bind to surrounding tissues. It can even encourage these unhealthy cells to create their own blood supply.

As it turns out, MCP naturally inhibits the effects of excess galectin-3 throughout the body. It does this by binding to this rogue protein molecule and blocking or neutralizing its undesirable effects.

MCP also promotes normal cell death function, and helps prevent the spread of poorly functioning cells. **It does this by a process called chelation.**

With chelation, MCP binds to the undesirable substance and you safely eliminate it during urination.

Key Benefits of EVERTO

- Supports Cellular Health
- Promotes Gentle Detoxification
- Supports Immune Health
- Modified for Enhanced Absorbability

Try EVERTO Now With a Special Offer

EVERTO supplies MCP — and a little extra fiber — in a tasty, chewable wafer. That makes it easy for your on-the-go lifestyle. No mixing or messy powders found with other typical products.

Medix Select is offering readers of Chelation Miracle a significant discount — as much as a 50% off Everto. Please do your cells and immune system a favor. Take advantage of a special discount on this powerful formula.

Learn How to Save 50% at:
MedixEverto.com/Miracle

More Titles From Humanix Books You May Be Interested In:

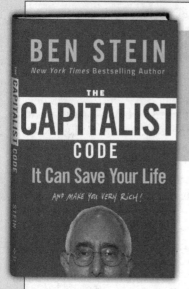

Warren Buffett says:

"My friend, Ben Stein, has written a short book that tells you everything you need to know about investing (and in words you can understand). Follow Ben's advice and you will do far better than almost all investors (and I include pension funds, universities and the super-rich) who pay high fees to advisors."

In his entertaining and informative style that has captivated generations, beloved *New York Times* bestselling author, actor, and financial expert Ben Stein sets the record straight about capitalism in the United States — it is not the "rigged system" young people are led to believe.

Dr. Mehmet Oz says:

"*SNAP!* shows that personalities can be changed from what our genes or early childhood would have ordained. Invest the 30 days."

New York Times bestselling author Dr. Gary Small's breakthrough plan to improve your personality for a better life! As you read *SNAP!* you will gain a better understanding of who you are now, how others see you, and which aspects of yourself you'd like to change. You will acquire the tools you need to change your personality in just one month — it won't take years of psychotherapy, self-exploration, or re-hashing every single bad thing that's ever happened to you.

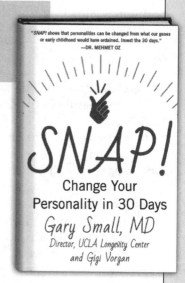

Get these books at Amazon and bookstores everywhere or checkout the FREE OFFERS! See:

www.HumanixBooks.com